PRAISE for **TRAUMA AND MEMORY**

"In yet another seminal work Peter Levine here deconstructs traumatic memory, making it accessible to healing and transformation. He helps us—therapist or client—move from a limiting past to where we belong: the empowered present."
—Gabor Maté, MD, author of *In the Realm of Hungry Ghosts: Close Encounters with Addiction* and *When the Body Says No: Exploring the Stress-Disease Connection*

"Arguably, much of our lives are spent at the mercy of the automatic brain; this is only accentuated for those who have experienced severe trauma. In writing with such depth and insight about the psychobiological dynamics of procedural memory, master therapist Peter Levine offers therapists important tools for the transformation of traumatic memory. Moreover, the writing and rich examples make this book accessible so that professionals and nonprofessionals alike can benefit from its wisdom."
—Stan Tatkin, PsyD, MFT, author of *Wired for Love*; founder of the PACT Institute

"With this book, Dr. Levine has made another significant contribution to the treatment of trauma. Drawing on established neuroscience he explains, in clear and accessible terms, the various kinds of memory, their neurological bases, and their role in the treatment of trauma. This book is invaluable for clinicians wishing to improve their skills, laypeople wanting a deeper understanding of the way the mind and brain work to create and heal trauma, and scientists looking to understand the implications of modern neuroscience for the treatment of trauma by the body-oriented psychotherapies."
—Peter Payne and Mardi Crane-Godreau, PhD, researchers at the Geisel School of Medicine at Dartmouth College

TRAUMA
AND
MEMORY

BRAIN AND BODY IN
A SEARCH FOR THE LIVING PAST

*A Practical Guide for
Understanding and Working
with Traumatic Memory*

PETER A. LEVINE, PhD

Foreword by Bessel A. Van der Kolk, MD

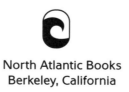

North Atlantic Books
Berkeley, California

Published by
North Atlantic Books
Berkeley, California

and

ERGOS Institute Press
P.O. Box 110
Lyons, Colorado 80540

Cover photo © Shutterstock.com/Volt Collection
Cover and book design by Howie Severson
Printed in the United States of America

Photos on pages 75–91 © Laura Regalbuto. All other photos and illustrations © Justin Snavely, except where noted.

Trauma and Memory: Brain and Body in a Search for the Living Past is sponsored and published by the Society for the Study of Native Arts and Sciences (dba North Atlantic Books), an educational nonprofit based in Berkeley, California, that collaborates with partners to develop cross-cultural perspectives, nurture holistic views of art, science, the humanities, and healing, and seed personal and global transformation by publishing work on the relationship of body, spirit, and nature.

North Atlantic Books' publications are available through most bookstores. For further information, visit our website at www.northatlanticbooks.com or call 800-733-3000.

Library of Congress Cataloging-in-Publication Data

Levine, Peter A., author.
  Trauma and memory : brain and body in a search for the living past : a practical guide for understanding and working with traumatic memory / Peter A. Levine.
      pages cm
  Summary: "Discusses different types of memory formation, especially traumatic memory, and how somatic or body-based memory can be utilized in the therapeutic process"— Provided by publisher.
  ISBN 978-1-58394-994-8 (paperback) — ISBN 978-1-58394-995-5 (ebook)
  1. Memory disorders. 2. Episodic memory. 3. Psychic trauma. 4. Post-traumatic stress disorder. I. Title.
  BF376.L48 2015
  153.1'3—dc23
                              2015023111

3 4 5 6 7 8 9 10 UNITED 20 19 18 17 16

Printed on recycled paper

Memory is the scribe of the soul.

—ARISTOTLE

Acknowledgments

In wrestling with the complex topic of traumatic memory, and making it comprehensible and practical, I offer my deep and special appreciation to Laura Regalbuto, my primary editor. Her contribution, however, goes well beyond that role, as she has many times challenged and nudged me in the direction of greater clarity, cohesion, and simplicity. Laura, you have been a partner and fellow traveler on this long road of discovery, understanding, and communication. To Justin Snavely, often working behind the scenes, I thank you for your fabulous technical assistance and help with the illustrations.

I wish to acknowledge my partners at North Atlantic Books, particularly Erin Wiegand, the project manager. And although we sometimes didn't agree on every editorial point, it was always a collaborative effort, infused with mutual good will and respect. Also, my appreciation to Lauren Harrison for her copyediting and the artistic staff at NAB, for their help on the cover design and layout.

Finally, to Richard Grossinger, the founder of North Atlantic Books: You have held to a lifelong vision of promoting high-caliber books on healing. I hope that you and NAB will continue in this independent and pioneering direction. Many of the books that were once considered "fringe" are now part of a revitalized mainstream, thanks in large part to your vision and commitment.

Contents

Foreword

The study of traumatic memories has a long and venerable pedigree in psychology and psychiatry. It goes back at least to Paris in the 1870s, when Jean-Martin Charcot, the father of neurology, became fascinated with the question of what caused the paralyses, jerky movements, swooning, sudden collapse, frenzied laughter, and dramatic weeping in the hysterical patients on the wards of the hospital of the Salpêtrière. Charcot and his students gradually came to understand that these bizarre movements and body postures were the physical imprints of trauma.

In 1889, Charcot's student Pierre Janet wrote the first book on what we now would call PTSD, *L'automatisme psychologique,** in which he argued that trauma is held in procedural memory—in automatic actions and reactions, sensations and attitudes, and that trauma is replayed and reenacted as visceral sensations (anxiety and panic), body movements, or visual images (nightmares and flashbacks). Janet put the issue of memory front and center in dealing with trauma: An event only becomes a trauma when overwhelming emotions interfere with proper memory processing. Afterward, traumatized patients react to reminders of the trauma with emergency responses appropriate to the original threat, but these reactions now are completely out of place—like ducking in panic under the table when a drinking glass falls on the floor, or going into a rage when a child starts crying.

For well over a century we have understood that the imprints of trauma are stored not as narratives about bad things that happened

---

* Pierre Janet, *L'automatisme psychologique: Essai de psychologie expérimentale sur les formes Inférieures de l'activité humaine* (Paris: Société Pierre Janet/Payot, 1973).

sometime in the past, but as physical sensations that are experienced as immediate life threats—*right now.* In the intervening time we have gradually come to understand that the difference between ordinary memories (stories that change and that fade with time) and traumatic memories (recurring sensations and movements that are accompanied by intense negative emotions of fear, shame, rage, and collapse) is the result of a breakdown of the brain systems that are responsible for creating "autobiographical memories."*

Janet also noted that traumatized people get stuck in the past: They become obsessed with the horror they consciously want to leave behind, but they keep behaving and feeling as if it is still going on. Unable to put the trauma behind them, their energy is absorbed by keeping their emotions under control at the expense of paying attention to the demands of the present. Janet and his colleagues learned from bitter experience that the traumatized women under their care could not be cured by reasoning or insight, behavior modification or punishment, but that they did respond to hypnotic suggestion: Trauma could be resolved by reliving the events in a hypnotic trance state. By safely replaying the old events in their minds and then constructing an imaginary satisfactory conclusion—something they had been unable to do during the original event because they had been too overwhelmed by helplessness and horror—they could begin to fully realize that they had, in fact, survived the trauma and could resume their lives.

When I first met Peter Levine about twenty-five years ago, I thought I had met a reincarnation of one of those old magicians whose work I knew so well from musty manuscripts that I found in the stacks of old hospital libraries. Except instead of wearing a bow tie and an evening frock customary in early photographs, Peter was dressed in a Bob Marley T-shirt and shorts, standing on the lawn

---

* Bessel van der Kolk, *The Body Keeps the Score: Brain, Mind, and Body in the Healing of Trauma* (New York: Viking, 2014).

of the Esalen Institute in Big Sur, California. Peter demonstrated he fully understood that trauma is imprinted in the body, and that in order to heal one needs to create a sheltered trance state from which one can safely observe the horrific past. And he added the critical element of exploring the subtle *physical* imprints of trauma and focused on reconnecting the body with the mind.

I was immediately intrigued. Starting with the earliest students of traumatic stress and continuing with the most recent neuroscience research, scientists have noted a critical relationship between bodily action and memory. An experience becomes traumatic when the human organism becomes overwhelmed and reacts with helplessness and paralysis—when there is absolutely nothing you can do to alter the outcome of events, the whole system comes crashing down. Even Sigmund Freud was fascinated by the relationship between trauma and physical action. He proposed that the reason people keep repeating their traumas is due to their inability to fully remember what has happened. Because the memory is repressed, the patient "is obliged to repeat the repressed material as a contemporary experience, instead of ... remembering it as something belonging to the past."* If a person does not remember, he is likely to act it out: "He reproduces it not as a memory but as an action; he *repeats* it, without, of course, knowing that he is repeating it ... in the end we understand that this is his way of remembering."† But the thing Freud did not realize was that people can only regain ownership over themselves if they can be helped to feel safe and calm inside.

Peter understood that in order to resolve trauma, you have to deal with physical paralysis, agitation and helplessness, and find

---

* Sigmund Freud, *Beyond the Pleasure Principle (The Standard Edition).* (New York: W. W. Norton & Company, 1990), 19.
† Sigmund Freud, "Remembering, Repeating, and Working Through." In *Standard Edition of the Complete Psychological Works, Vol. XII.* (New York: W. W. Norton & Company, 1990), 150.

some way of taking *bodily* action to regain ownership of your life. Even telling the story of what has happened is a form of effective action, developing a narrative that allows you and those around you to know what has happened. Sadly, numerous traumatized people become stuck in their trauma and never have a chance to develop that essential narrative.

As I got to know Peter better, I gradually realized how well he understood the critical role of physical sensations and bodily action. He showed that post-traumatic actions do not only consist of gross behaviors such as blowing up at anyone who offends you or becoming paralyzed when you are scared, but also in imperceptibly holding your breath, tensing your muscles, or tightening your sphincters. He showed me that the entire organism—body, mind, and spirit—becomes stuck and continues to behave as if there is a clear and present danger. Peter was originally trained as a neurophysiologist and then studied bodywork at Esalen with Ida Rolf. When I witnessed him exercising his craft, I was reminded of Moshe Feldenkrais, who claimed that there are no purely psychic (i.e., mental) experiences: "The idea of two lives, somatic and psychic, has … outlived its usefulness."* Our subjective experience always has a bodily component, just as all so-called bodily experiences have a mental component.

The brain is programmed by mental experiences that are expressed in the body. Emotions are communicated in facial expressions and body postures: Anger is experienced by clenched fists and gritted teeth; fear is rooted in tightened muscles and shallow breath. Thoughts and emotions are accompanied by changes in our muscle tension, and in order to change habitual patterns one has to change the somatic loops that connect sensations, thoughts, memories, and actions. The primary task of therapists then is to observe and deal with those somatic changes.

---

* Moshe Feldenkrais, *Body and Mature Behavior.* (Berkeley: North Atlantic Books, 2005), 191.

When I was a student at the University of Chicago, Eugene Gendlin tried to teach me about "the felt sense"—the awareness of one's self, the space between thought and action—but I didn't fully appreciate what the felt sense was until I witnessed Peter utilizing physical awareness as the key to learning. His use of touch helped me enormously. Touch had been strictly prohibited in my training and sorely neglected in my upbringing, but Peter's use of touch helped me become more aware of my inner experiences and made me understand the enormous power of touch to help people borrow comfort and physiological safety from each other.

Becoming aware of inner sensations, our primordial feelings, allows us access to the direct experience of our own living body along a scale that ranges from pleasure to pain, feelings that originate at the deepest levels of the brain stem rather than the cerebral cortex. This is so important to understand, because traumatized people are terrified of what's going on inside of them. Asking them to focus on their breath may precipitate a panic reaction; simply requesting that they keep still often only increases their agitation.

We can observe the neural corollary of this alienation from the physical self in brain scans: The areas of the brain that are devoted to self-awareness (the medial prefrontal cortex) and body awareness (the insula) often are shrunk in people with chronic PTSD—the body/mind/brain has learned to shut itself down. This shutting down carries an enormous price: The same brain areas that convey pain and distress are also responsible for transmitting feelings of joy, pleasure, purpose, and relational connection.

Peter showed me, and shows us in this book, how negative judgment of oneself or others causes minds and bodies to tense up, which renders learning impossible. In order to recover, people need to feel free to explore and learn new ways to move. Only then can nervous systems reorganize themselves and new patterns be formed. This can only be done by investigating new ways of moving, breathing, and engaging, and cannot be accomplished by prescribing specific actions geared at "fixing."

In the chapters that follow, Peter Levine explains how traumatic memories are implicit, and are carried in body and brain as a patchwork of sensations, emotions, and behaviors. Traumatic imprints stealthily force themselves on us, not so much as stories or conscious memories, but as emotions, sensations, and "procedures"—things that the body automatically does, as psychological automatisms. If trauma is played out in procedural automatisms, healing cannot not be accomplished by advice, drugs, understanding, or fixing, but rather by accessing the inborn life force (my word), which Peter calls "our innate drive for perseverance and triumph."

What does this consist of? Getting to know yourself, feeling your physical impulses, noticing how your body stiffens and contracts, and how emotions, memories, and impulses arise as the awareness of your interiority increases. Sensory imprints of trauma can have powerful effects on our subsequent reactions, behaviors, and emotional feeling states. After having become accustomed to constantly be on guard against letting these demons from the past enter our consciousness, we must instead learn to simply notice them without judgment and observe them for what they are: signals to activate inborn motor action programs. Following their natural course will help rearrange our relationship to ourselves. However, this mindful self-surveillance is easily overwhelmed, which precipitates panic, explosive actions, freezing, or collapse.

One of the fundamental concepts to deal with this sensitivity to fall apart is Peter's notion of "pendulation": touching on your inner sensations and learning to tolerate them by noticing that you will survive feeling them, but to then deliberately return to safer routines. This work is not about abreaction, or, as I like to call it, "vomiting out your trauma." Learning to carefully access "the felt sense" opens up the possibility of getting to know the danger signals that lurk deep inside and to gain mastery over them. Before it is safe to feel the sensations associated with terror and annihilation you first have to get in touch with what inner strength and healthy aggression feel like.

One of the most brilliant and original discussions in this book is Peter's explanation of how, in order to meet extreme adversity, one needs to engage both the brain's motivation and action systems. The motivation system is run by the brain's dopamine system, and the action system by the noradrenergic system. In order to meet great challenges with a sense of purpose, both need to be galvanized in the therapeutic process. These are necessary conditions for confronting and transforming the demons of the past from helpless surrender to competent self-ownership.

Good therapy consists of learning to call up the felt sense without becoming overwhelmed by what's lurking inside. The most important sentences in any therapy are "notice that" and "notice what happens next." Allowing yourself to observe your inner processes activates brain pathways that connect the rational and the emotional parts of the brain, and *this is the only known pathway through which a person can consciously rearrange the perceptual system of the brain.* In order to be in touch with your self, you have to activate the anterior insula, the critical brain area responsible for how you feel about your body and your self. Levine points out that most spiritual traditions have developed breathing, movement, and meditative techniques to facilitate tolerating and integrating deep emotional and sensory states.

Somatic Experiencing's slow, meticulous, mindful attention to inner sensations and subtle movements is very different from most expressive therapies that usually are focused on outwardly directed action rather than the felt sense of self. Attention to internal experiences uncovers procedural movements that tend to be unintentional and reflexive, and that probably engage different brain systems, like the cerebellum and extrapyramidal system, than intentional, willed actions do.

This work also stands in sharp contrast with therapeutic approaches that encourage survivors to repetitively relive their traumas in great detail and that run the risk of creating conditions under which traumatized individuals are kept in a state of high fear and physiological arousal, in which the agony of the past may well be reinforced. If that happens, the traumatic memory may become reconsolidated in association with those novel states of terror and only increase the sense of being overwhelmed by one's inner world.

This book is full of case histories and detailed accounts of how to put the principles of Somatic Experiencing into action, not only with victims of traumas such as car accidents, but also with neonates, toddlers, school-aged children, and combat soldiers. Somatic Experiencing is not primarily about "unlearning" conditioned responses to trauma by rehashing them, but about creating novel experiences that contradict overwhelming feelings of helplessness and replacing them with a sense of ownership of physical reactions and sensations.

This work lays the frozen shame, grief, rage, and sense of loss to rest by helping trauma's explosive assault on the body to be completed and resolved. Peter's work helps us transcend what he calls "the destructive explanation compulsion" and to create an inner sense of ownership and control over previously out-of-control sensations and reactions. In order to do that, we need to create an experience of embodied action, as opposed to helpless capitulation or uncontrollable rage. *Only after we become capable of standing back, taking stock of ourselves, reducing the intensity of our sensations and emotions, and activating our inborn physical defensive reactions can we learn to modify our entrenched maladaptive automatic survival responses and, in doing so, put our haunting memories to rest.*

—Bessel A. van der Kolk, MD
Cabot, Vermont, July 26, 2015

Lay of the Land

There is no present or future,
only the past, happening over and over again.
—Eugene O'Neill

The Tyranny of the Past

Throughout the ages people have been tormented by memories that have filled them with fright and horror, with feelings of helplessness, rage, hatred, and revenge, and with a plaguing sense of irreparable loss. In ancient literature, such as the epic tragedies of the Greeks, Sumerians, and Egyptians, as well as in hundreds of contemporary books on trauma, nightly newscasts, and celebrity confessionals, trauma has been and continues to be at the epicenter of human experience.

Despite the seemingly boundless human predilection to inflict suffering and trauma on others, we are also capable of surviving, adapting to, and eventually transforming traumatic experiences. Seasoned therapists utilize this innate capacity for resilience and healing to support their work with those suffering from the aftermath of life-threatening and overwhelming events. These incidents include (but are by no means limited to) war, assault, molestation, abuse, accidents, invasive medical procedures, natural disasters, and witnessing a serious injury or sudden death of a loved one. All of these "shocks" to the organism can alter a person's biological, psychological, and social equilibrium to such a degree that the memory of one particular event comes to taint, and dominate, all other experiences, spoiling an appreciation of the present moment. The resulting *tyranny of the past* interferes with the ability to focus effectively on both new and familiar situations. When people pay selective attention to the riveting reminders of their past, sleep becomes the enemy and life becomes colorless.

Perhaps nowhere in the field of trauma is there more confusion than with the role of traumatic memory in both pathology and healing. Indeed, research studies conducted by different laboratories frequently appear to contradict one another. In addition, clinicians and academics rarely communicate with each other—a very unfortunate state of affairs. Most importantly, traumatic memory differs fundamentally from other types of memory, creating the potential for great confusion and the misapplication of therapeutic techniques.

While this book is geared toward therapists who work with their clients' traumatic memories, it is also written for individuals trying to make sense of their own haunting memories and who long to know how they might come to an enduring peace with them. It is also for those avid readers who are simply interested in the scientific and clinical study of how memory plays out in the governance of their lives, its great ambiguities, its perplexing uncertainties, and what it takes to make sense of it all.

We begin this exploration with an understanding that memory exists in many forms—forms that fundamentally differ in both structure and function. At the same time, these distinct memory systems (involving different parts of the brain) must operate cooperatively to promote effective functioning and well-being. This book is about how we can learn to befriend our hauntings and liberate ourselves from their tyranny.

Most contemporary psychotherapies live in the long shadow cast by Freud and his descendants, or have been guided by various cognitive behavioral approaches. However, these avenues of alleviating human suffering are of limited value in work with trauma and its underlying memory imprints. While both of these therapeutic traditions do address certain dysfunctions related to trauma, they are unable to reach its primal core. They do not sufficiently address the essential body and brain mechanisms that are impacted by trauma. Alas, this leaves the most basic human need and drive for healing largely unmet.

Trauma shocks the brain, stuns the mind, and freezes the body. It overwhelms its unfortunate victims and hurls them adrift in a raging sea of torment, helplessness, and despair. For a therapist, to witness such desperation in one's clients is to feel a compelling call to effectively relieve such suffering. Increasingly, therapists are being drawn to work with traumatic memories as various techniques (and their offshoots) are becoming widely known, taught, and practiced. These various approaches have arrived on the scene in this approximate chronological order: mesmerism, hypnosis, analysis, exposure, Somatic Experiencing (SE), eye movement desensitization reprocessing (EMDR), and various "energy psychologies" (e.g., point tapping).

Many psychodynamic therapists understand that they must work with how their patients' pasts play out in the present. In this way they attempt to help them secure a better, healthier, more focused, effective, and vibrant future. However, without a working understanding of how trauma becomes inscribed as memory imprints in body, brain, and mind, as well as in psyche and soul, the healer is sure to lose his or her way in the labyrinth of cause and effect. For effective therapy, it is critical to appreciate just how trauma becomes riveted in the body's instinctive reactions to perceived threat; how it becomes fixated in certain emotions, particularly those of fear, terror, and rage, as well as in habitual affective mood states such as depression, bipolarity, and loss of vital energy; and finally, how it plays out in various self-destructive and repetitive behaviors.

Without a firm grasp of the *multidimensional structure of traumatic memory as it is stored in the brain and held in the body*, the therapist is often left floundering in the swamplands of ambiguity and uncertainty. Indeed, misconceptions about so-called recovered memories have caused much unnecessary pain and suffering for patients and for their families, while also creating confusion and self-doubt for the therapists who treat them.

Perhaps more than we might wish to admit, many therapists are influenced by common misconceptions about the nature of memory. Traditionally, both academic and clinical psychologists have tended to study what has been called "verbally accessible memory." This "declarative" form of memory is called upon and rewarded in elementary, middle, and high school, as well as in undergraduate and graduate studies. No small wonder then that psychologists and psychotherapists, as products of academia, tend to reflexively identify with this particular kind of conscious memory. However, conscious, *explicit* memory is only the proverbial tip of a very deep and mighty iceberg. It barely hints at the submerged strata of *primal implicit experience* that moves and motivates us in ways that the conscious mind can only begin to imagine. But imagine we should, and understand we must, if we are to work effectively and wisely with trauma and its memory traces in both mind and body.

MEMORY: GIFT AND CURSE

The Illusion of Memory

Memory is the selection of images; some elusive; others printed indelibly on the brain. Each image is like a thread … each thread woven together to make a tapestry of intricate textures. And the tapestry tells a story. And the story is our past … Like others before me, I have the gift of sight. But the truth changes color depending on the light. And tomorrow can be clearer than yesterday.
—EVE'S BAYOU, SCREENPLAY BY KASI LEMMONS

In early 2015, Brian Williams, a highly respected journalist and broadcast media star, retreated in shame and defeat over "lying" and inflating his exposure to extreme threat in his warfront coverage. We now know these facts: Williams was flying behind a helicopter that had been hit by a rocket-propelled grenade. Over time, his story mutated to a version where he recounted that he was riding in the helicopter that came under fire. Public and pundits alike were astonished that he would risk his reputation with such specious heroism and self-aggrandizement. We all asked ourselves how we could have been duped by this sincere and earnest reporter.

Yet consider other similar "missteps" by public figures: Hillary Rodham Clinton once claimed that she was under sniper fire in Bosnia, only to later admit that she "had her facts wrong." Not to be partisan, let us not forget that Mitt Romney remembered a Detroit jubilee that took place nine months before he was born! Are all of these notables outright liars, or is something else going on? The real answer is that these kinds of memory distortions, particularly when laid down in times of high stress and danger, are something to which we are all readily susceptible. On a lighter note, we can identify with Romney's "pre-birth memories," as many of us have incorporated a family photo or oft-repeated story into our "factually recalled" personal reminiscences. Indeed, the meaning we attach to a particular event can have a significant effect on the content of that memory. In the words of the psychoanalyst Alfred Adler: "Out of the incalculable number of impressions which meet an individual, he chooses to remember those which he feels, however darkly, to have a bearing on his situation."

Aristotle believed that humans are born as a tabula rasa—a blank slate—and that we are the product of a life imprinted as a series of memories, just as an impression is made in wax. However, memory is no such thing; we must live with the uncomfortable acceptance that memory is simply not something concrete, definitive, and reproducible, like a video recording that can be retrieved at will. It is instead more ephemeral, ever-shifting in shape and meaning. Memory is not a discrete phenomenon, a fixed construction, cemented permanently onto a stone foundation. Rather, it is more like a fragile house of cards, perched precariously upon the shifting sands of time, at the mercy of interpretation and confabulation. Indeed, memory is a continual reconstruction, more akin to the wayward, wildly unpredictable electrons in Heisenberg's uncertainty principle. Just as the very act of observing electrons changes their position or momentum, so does the warp and woof of memory interweave to yield a soft fabric that changes hue and contour with the movement of light and shadow throughout the day and over the seasons.

Literature and film have long been fascinated by the fallacies of memory. The fragility and inherent subjectivity of memory are brilliantly portrayed in Akira Kurosawa's 1950 film *Rashomon*, in which four characters each recall their starkly contrasting memories of the same event. Just as in the movie, memory is like a fleeting dream: Just as one tries to grasp it, memory slips away, leaving us with the stark consolation that the ever-changing eye of the beholder may be the only truly reliable defining quality of recollection. So can we observe our memories without changing them in the process of recall? The short answer is no.

Philosophers and filmmakers, along with a growing number of contemporary cognitive neuroscientists, question the validity of recollection per se. Mark Twain once confessed, "I am an old man and I have known a great number of misfortunes, but most of them never happened." In other words, his immediate and current misery caused him to "remember" (i.e., construct) events that never really happened. Indeed, recent research resoundingly demonstrates that memory is a *reconstructive process* that is continuously selecting, adding, deleting, rearranging, and updating information—all to serve the ongoing adaptive process of survival and living.

In the following chapters we'll explore the implications of the mutability of memory, as well as pursue an understanding of the types of memory that pertain specifically to trauma. A central premise to be explored in this work is that our present feeling state may be the major factor determining what and how we remember a particular event. Indeed, first changing our current feeling state is a sine qua non for effective work with traumatic memories. What has been poorly understood in clinical work with traumatic memories is that our present mood, emotions, and somatic sensations (generated for whatever reasons) profoundly influence what we are "remembering." Remembered images and thoughts that appear in our field of awareness are evoked and (unconsciously) selected to match our current emotional state. Our current moods and sensations play a key role in *how* we remember a particular event—they structure our evolving relationship to these "memories," as well as how we deal with and reconstruct them anew.

The key to investigating the utility and reliability of memory lies in studying its biological roots, together with its psychological, developmental, and social functions. If memory proves to be decidedly elusive and illusive, then what is its value, and what are its inherent limitations? When can a memory be trusted and when will it betray, leaving us floundering in a sea of ambiguity and uncertainty? Furthermore, when is the memory a fabrication perpetrated by "magicians," be they therapists, family, lawyers, or politicians? When might it be a twisted distortion of history fostered by the collective unconscious of societies, tribes, or clans? And when are the actions of these sorcerers and forces deliberate, and when are they unwitting?

With regard to transforming trauma, many therapeutic modalities seem to misunderstand or even ignore the essential questions: Under which conditions might a memory be a healing force and when might it be destructive? When might it generate self-inflicted pain and unnecessary suffering? Ultimately, and most importantly, how can we tell the difference?

A Walk Down Memory Lane

Memories form the very bedrock of our identities and help define what it means to be human. Though not necessarily entirely accurate or permanent, memories are a magnetic compass that guides us through new situations. They help us render a *context* for these emerging experiences so that we are able to confidently plan our next steps while developing coherent stories about our life's trajectory. It is, in short, via memories that we find our way in the world. Problems and difficulties that arise when taking up new hobbies, learning new dance steps, connecting with strangers, and understanding new concepts can be directly correlated to our lack of previously established templates around which we organize new information and new experiences.

Memory, when reduced to its most vital function, has to do with securing a future that chooses *selectively* from the past and builds on what was effective, while not repeating those responses that were deleterious or harmful—in short, securing a future that is influenced, but not overly constrained, by our history. Through memory we maintain a thread of continuity by linking present with past. In the ongoing process of comparing similarities and differences, times of threat and those of safety and contentment, as well as important accomplishments and failures, we sort through and then reorganize this information to shape our present and upcoming choices. In this way we aspire to create a future more adaptive, rewarding, and beneficial than our past. The words of the country singer Vince Gill ring true: There simply "ain't no future in the past."

Memories, such as the recollection of a wonderful walk in the woods on a crisp and colorful day while kicking piles of leaves into the air and sharing intimate thoughts and feelings with a close friend, are pleasantly welcomed back into the folds of our consciousness. Though sometimes distant, these reminiscences are often infused with faint sensory impressions such as the musty scent of the leaves or the crackling sounds as they are kicked aloft, the cool nip in the air or the exquisite colors of autumn foliage. Just as familiar are unpleasant memories from which we recoil and would prefer to forget. These negative recollections are often very powerful in seizing our attention. When, for example, we are rejected by a lover or passed over for a promotion, we cannot get these events out of our minds. And, indeed, they may linger, pungent and poignant, for years, sometimes seeming to have the same bite when they are recalled as when they first happened. Any smells, sights, sounds, and sensations associated with these memories can be disturbing, distasteful, aggravating, or even repellant. Such responses compel avoidance of voluntary and subconscious contact with any reminders. Nonetheless, we may find ourselves sharing these painful reminiscences with friends or therapists as relatively sensible and coherent stories—whether describing pleasurable or disturbing past experiences. We are usually able to reflect on these memories, learn something from them, and move forward with our lives. We are potentially enriched and empowered by our mistakes and failures, as well as by our great or little triumphs and achievements.

The most salient of our memories are imbued with sensations and feelings, whether good or bad, joyful or sad, angry or content. It is, in fact, the emotional impact associated with a memory that is largely responsible for initiating and strengthening learning. Indeed, what we call learning is actually a process of importing the patterns, affects, behaviors, perceptions, and constructs recorded from previous experiences (i.e., "memory engrams"[1]) to meet the demands of current encounters. In short, past imprints influence present and future planning, often under the radar of conscious awareness. In contrast to a repetitive news clip, our memories are mutable, molded and remolded many times throughout our lives. They are continuously in flux, perpetually in a process of forming and reforming.

Traumatic Memory

No worst, there is none.
—GERARD MANLEY HOPKINS

In contrast to "ordinary" memories (both good and bad), which are mutable and dynamically changing over time, traumatic memories are fixed and static. They are imprints (engrams) from past overwhelming experiences, deep impressions carved into the sufferer's brain, body, and psyche. These harsh and frozen imprints do not yield to change, nor do they readily update with current information. The "fixity" of imprints prevents us from forming new strategies and extracting new meanings. There is no fresh, ever-changing now and no real flow in life. In this way, *the past lives on in the present*; or as William Faulkner wrote in *Requiem for a Nun*: "The past is never dead. It's not even past." Rather, it lives as a panoply of manifold fears, phobias, physical symptoms, and illnesses.

In sharp contrast to gratifying or even troublesome memories, which can generally be formed and revisited as coherent narratives, "traumatic memories" tend to arise as fragmented splinters of inchoate and indigestible sensations, emotions, images, smells, tastes, thoughts, and so on. For example, a motorist who survived a fiery car crash is suddenly besieged by a racing heart, stark terror, and a desperate need to flee when he catches a whiff of gasoline while filling his tank at a service station. These jumbled fragments cannot be remembered in the narrative sense per se, but are perpetually being "replayed" and re-experienced as unbidden and incoherent intrusions or physical symptoms. The more we try to rid ourselves of these "flashbacks," the more they haunt, torment, and strangle our life force, seriously restricting our capacity to live in the here and now.

Traumatic memories may also take the form of unconscious "acting-out" behaviors. These include, for example, repeatedly having "accidents" or unwittingly exposing oneself to dangerous situations. A couple of cases in point are the prostitute who, molested as a child, now seeks liaisons with violent men or has unprotected sex; or the war vet, "addicted" to thrill and danger, who applies for the police SWAT team immediately after discharge from the military.

"Relived" traumatic memories erupt involuntarily as raw tatters of experience, suddenly imposing themselves on the vulnerable sufferer. These shards seem to come out of nowhere, cutting into their victims' lives, whether waking or sleeping. To be traumatized is to be condemned to an endless nightmare, replaying these unbearable torments, as well as being prey to various obsessions and compulsions. Traumatized people have their lives arrested until they are somehow able to process these intrusions, assimilate them, and then finally form coherent narratives that help put these memories to rest; or said another way, to come to peace with their memories. This *completion* restores continuity between past and future, and prompts a motivating perseverance and a realistic optimism and forward movement in life.

Looking Back

The role of trauma memories in the treatment of "neurosis" was the Rosetta stone of early twentieth-century psychoanalysis. While Freud was hardly the first to deal with such pathogenic and hidden ("repressed") memories, he became the best known. In truth, he stood tall on the broad shoulders of giants who came before him, notably Jean-Martin Charcot and Pierre Janet working at the Salpêtrière in Paris. They really were the first to appreciate how traumatic memory can be walled off from consciousness by the mechanisms of what they called repression and dissociation, and then how therapy consisted of bringing these split-off parts into conscious awareness. Their pioneering contribution must have been an inspiration to Freud, influencing his early trauma theory.

However, as Freud abandoned the recognition of trauma's origin in overwhelming (external) events and turned to the internal machinations of the "Oedipal" and other "instinctual conflicts," Janet's great contribution was eclipsed. With Freud's charismatic dominance, and the messy reality of familial abuse and molestation, trauma from overwhelming external events all but disappeared from the radar of psychology—that is, until the "shell shocked" soldiers of World War I returned home. Society and psychology preferred to follow Freud's new focus on internal conflicts (such as the "Oedipal complex"), while veering away from the murky and disturbing family dynamics of childhood sexual abuse, perpetrated even in the Victorian homes of respectable doctors, lawyers, and bankers. Fortunately, Janet's profound understanding of trauma, its etiology, and its implications for treatment were revisited some hundred years later by Bessel van der Kolk and Onno van der Hart in a seminal paper celebrating the centenary of Janet's landmark book, *L'automatisme psychologique*, first published in 1889.[2,3] This foundational history in the understanding and treatment of trauma is elegantly treated and respectfully honored in van der Kolk's recent comprehensive book *The Body Keeps the Score*.

Memory Wars: The Truth about False Memories, the Falsity of True Memories, and the Unholy Grail of "Memory Erasure"

Memory is the historical accumulation of lies …
Like memory, good fiction must have specific dates
and times; that way it seems to be true.
—Daniel Schmid, Swiss film director

At the turn of the twenty-first century, memory had become the elusive Holy Grail of contemporary cognitive neuroscience, snagging a Nobel Prize for Physiology in 2000.* In contrast, fifteen years earlier, the pivotal role of memory in the treatment of trauma had fostered a violent schism, a virtual memory war. On one side of this highly polarized clash were therapists who vehemently pushed their clients to "recover" long-forgotten, "dissociated," or "repressed" memories of childhood molestation and abuse. This agonizing dredging was generally accompanied by repeated dramatic abreactions† and often by violent catharsis. These highly charged, "expressive" therapies were frequently carried out in group settings where participants were encouraged (or often pressured) to scream out their anguish and rage as they "recovered" horrific memory after horrific memory.

Many of these patients were female college students suffering from depression, anxiety, and panic disorders who were desperate to discover a cause, and in doing so, find a cure for their suffering. Their crippling anguish made them frantic to find a denouement, an absolution, in the temporary relief afforded by these intense abreactions. The perceived veracity of these "recovered" memories helped them to "explain" to themselves and to find an anchor for their states of profound distress. These catharses also stimulated the release of highly addictive rushes of adrenaline and a flood of endogenous opioids (endorphins).[4] This biochemical cocktail, along with the potent group bonding (also opioid mediated) derived from the sharing of similar stories, was powerfully

---

* Eric Kandel won the prize for his studies of learning in the giant axon-synapse of the sea slug (Aplysia).

† *Abreaction* refers to a method in which one becomes conscious of and "relives" a traumatic event that has been repressed.

compelling.[5] Indeed, many of these sufferers did have family histories of abuse and horrors that were being uncovered by these therapies. Unfortunately, they were often confused or inaccurate. And even when accurate, they frequently did not provide deep and enduring healing. In many cases, this dredging caused great amounts of unnecessary suffering. Many of the guiding therapists believed, wholly and completely, in the veracity and therapeutic value of these "recovered" memories, even if that meant sometimes believing things that could not possibly have happened, as well as denying the deleterious effects of the so-called recovery on the lives of patients and their families.

On the other side of this developing skirmish was a group of academic memory researchers who were just as vehement in their assertion that these "recovered" memories were often false—that they were confabulations. They based this conclusion largely on experiments in which they had successfully implanted "traumatic" memories of events that were verifiably false. The most impressive of these experiments involved getting college subjects to believe deliberately implanted false memories of being lost in a mall as a small child. These "memories" often included clear images of being found by a stranger and then being taken to their parents. However, prior interviews with the students' parents had confirmed that events like these never actually took place. In a rebuttal of this experiment, Bessel van der Kolk points out that the student subjects did not exhibit the visceral distress that would most certainly have accompanied remembering such a terrifying childhood episode.[6] Nonetheless, experiments like this led many memory researchers to conclude that many, if not most, therapeutically recovered memories were subconsciously implanted by unwitting—or in some cases willful—therapists. But first, the telling story of Beth.

Beth

It was under suspicious circumstances that the mother of thirteen-year-old Beth was found dead, drowned in the family swimming pool. The grief-stricken teen must have also been tormented by the possibility that her mother had taken her own life. Two years after this devastating shock, Beth also lost her home. A brush fire destroyed the house while sparing others on her block.

Imagine the stunned, motherless girl standing outside her burning home, holding a ragged teddy bear close to her chest. According to one report, she was particularly troubled by the disappearance of her diary. Her biggest fear was not that it was lost in the fire but rather that it might fall into another person's hands.[7] One can only imagine what memories and private secrets this vulnerable adolescent shared with her diary.

What did Beth make of all this loss? How did she deal with the lurking presence of these haunting ghosts? How had she managed the ambiguity of her mother's death followed by the sudden destruction of her family's home? Like the contents of her diary, we will never know these answers. And yet, in time, the direction of Beth's adult life came to tell its own revealing story of courage, fortitude, perseverance, and concentrated focus: Elizabeth Loftus grew up to become a renowned expert on memory.

For years, Professor Loftus crusaded against recovered memory therapies, obsessed with proving that many of these therapeutically evoked abuse memories are false. She then began a determined inquiry into the possibility of memory erasure with research on student attitudes concerning the elimination of disturbing memories. Undergraduates were asked whether they would want to take a memory-dampening drug in the event that they had been mugged and beaten. Nearly half stated that they would want the right to access such a drug. However, only 14 percent said they would actually use it.[8] In a similar inquiry, only 20 percent of a group of firefighters who were "Ground Zero" rescuers at the World Trade Center on September 11, 2001, said they would want a pill to erase their horrific memories. To say that Professor Loftus was surprised by this data would certainly be an understatement. In her own words, she asserted that, "If I had endured an assault I would take the drug."[9] Indeed, although she doesn't seem to have quite made the connection, Beth had, of course, actually undergone an "assault" with the wrenching losses of her mother and her childhood home.

No matter how much a hurt child, like young Beth, wants to flee from her memories, they will still trail after her, insidious ghosts lurking in the shadows. Who wouldn't want to eradicate these hauntings from the vaults of their memory banks? But, one wonders, at what risk and at what cost to our unique humanness? We shall discover that there are more constructive and life-affirming ways to approach and engage our difficult memories.

Painful memories shape our lives in ways we might not ever suspect. Like the many-headed Hydra (and our beleaguered futile fight to cut off head after head), these memories will come back to bite us, haunt us, and mold us, no matter how much we aspire to eliminate, deny, or sanctify them. How might we work *with* rather than *against* them, accessing and utilizing their "compressed energy" to liberate us from their stranglehold?

Let us recognize that ultimately, both views of memory, false or recovered, are off the mark, particularly with regard to the role of memory in healing trauma and other wounds of the psyche and soul. Both camps and their remedies are arguably slamming into their own unresolved traumas, psychodynamic issues, scientific biases, prejudices, and the "cherry-picking" of data to support their hardened positions. It is as though each group sees the other side as inherently dishonest or worse, and assumes that all of their beliefs and data are automatically wrong, even when the research or clinical observations were carried out methodically and rendered results consistent with other data. Both groups seem unnecessarily defensive and profoundly unwilling to learn from each other. Unfortunately, their differences have played out not in the halls of science, objectivity, and open inquiry, but rather in the courts of law, tabloid "journalism," and public opinion—often via the stories of media celebrities.

Even more fundamental to these "memory wars" is the broad misunderstanding about the very nature of memory itself.

2

THE FABRIC OF MEMORY

Memories are made of this ...

To comprehend the nature of traumatic memory, it is necessary to step back from the precipitous brink of the "memory wars" and begin to tease out the various component strands that when woven together form the multi-textured fabric of what we call "memory." Broadly speaking, there are two types of memory: those that are *explicit* and those that are *implicit,* the former being conscious and the latter relatively unconscious. These two memory systems—each of which has at least two broad subcategories—serve separate functions and are mediated by distinct neuro-anatomical brain structures. At the same time, they are meant to guide us (see Figure 2.1) as we navigate life's various situations and challenges.

Explicit Memory: Declarative and Episodic

Well, I do declare!
—SCARLETT O'HARA, *GONE WITH THE WIND*

Declarative memories are the most familiar subtype of explicit memory. They are a catalogue of detailed data, the laundry and shopping lists of the memory world. Declarative memories allow us to consciously remember things and to tell reasonably factual stories about them, stories with beginnings, middles, and ends. Most lay persons, as well as many therapists, tend to think of memory primarily as this concrete form. It is only this one reified type of memory that we can actively and deliberately call up or declare. The general role of declarative memories is to communicate discrete pieces of information to other individuals. These "semantic" memories are objective and devoid of feelings and emotions. Without declarative memory there would be no cars, airplanes, computers, email, smartphones, bicycles, skateboards, or even pens. Indeed, there would be no books. Without it, fire probably wouldn't have been utilized and spread throughout the world, and we would still be helplessly huddled in damp, dark caves. In short, civilization as we know it wouldn't exist.

Declarative memories are relatively orderly, neat, and tidy, like the highly structured cerebral cortex that they use for their hardware and operating system. While declarative memories are the most conscious and voluntary of the memory systems, they are, by far, the least compelling and enlivening. For the purpose of in-depth psychodynamic approaches, declarative memories are, by themselves, rarely therapeutically relevant. Yet in contrast, they are the basic component of many cognitive and behavioral interventions.

If declarative memory is characterized as "cold" factual information, *episodic memory*—a second form of explicit memory—would be, in contrast, "warm" and textured. Episodic memories are often infused with feeling tones and vitality, whether of positive or negative valence, and richly encode our personal life experiences. They form a dynamic interface between the "rational" (explicit/declarative) and "irrational" (implicit/emotional) realms. This intermediary function promotes the formation of coherent narratives, the poignant stories that we tell to ourselves and others and which help

Types of Memory

Explicit   **Implicit**

⟋ ⟍   ⟋ ⟍
Declarative   Episodic   Emotional   Procedural
                                           ("Body Memory")

Most Conscious		Least Conscious

Figure 2.1. Basic Memory Systems

us make sense of our lives. The linking and processing of raw emotion, nuanced feeling, fact, and communication with chosen others is essential in moving from trauma—with a future barely different from the past—to an open future built upon new experiences, information, and possibilities.

Remembrance of Things Past

Episodic memory (sometimes called autobiographical), rather than being called up deliberately, emerges somewhat spontaneously as representative vignettes from our lives. These memories generally convey a vague feeling tone, often infused with a dreamlike quality. On the awareness hierarchy, these autobiographical reminiscences are less conscious than the "shopping list" type of declarative memories, but more conscious—as we shall see—than implicit memories. In general, episodic memories have more felt nuance and an oblique capacity for ambiguity than do the declarative (factual) memories. When we focus our attention in their general direction, we can hazily drift with episodic memories, in and out of recollection. While these memories are sometimes indistinct and vague, they may in other instances have an eidetic, vivid, lifelike quality. Episodic memories are more spontaneous, interesting, and enlivening than the "laundry list" declarative ones. They frequently have an important, though often subterranean, influence on our lives.

A personal example of an episodic memory is the recollection I have of walking home from my first day of fifth grade at P.S. 94 in the Bronx. I remember talking with my friends about how *terrible* my new teacher was. A gentle tap on my right shoulder interrupted the drone of my exaggerated and premature grievances. My stomach dropped as I turned to see the gray-haired Mrs. Kurtz. "Do you think I am really *that* bad?" she queried, tipping her head as she eyed me quizzically. This story had a happy ending, as Mrs. Kurtz turned out to be the best teacher I had in elementary school, and I welcome this episodic memory back with a quality of rueful fondness. And though I would be hard-pressed to recall anything else about my fifth grade year, this recollection somehow encapsulates and represents that entire turnaround year for me. It certainly doesn't twist my gut as it did then when I first felt her hand on my shoulder.

As mentioned before, in looking back on that year, other than this one memory of Mrs. Kurtz, I have almost no voluntary recall. Indeed, I have only a few scattered memories from grades one through six, and most of those are very unpleasant. All of my other teachers were singularly uninspiring, and some were even cruel and sadistic. Rather than embodying the Latin root for education (*educare*: to bring up or to draw out), my basic grade school experience ("model") of education was that of having subjects shoved down my gullet. I hated school and school hated me!

The episodic memory of Mrs. Kurtz evolved into a substantive part of my personal, autobiographical narrative. It became the way I understand, and tell others about, this period in my life. Though initially hidden from me, the memory of Mrs. Kurtz came to function as a kind of pivot, an inflection point, away from an otherwise oppressive, dreary "learning" experience. It catalyzed the creation of a new composite memory, one where learning could be positive and even fun. This allowed for a newly felt belief system, one that extended through my future education and into today's vocation and avocations.

After the fifth grade and through high school (a dangerous and violent place, rampant with knife-wielding Bronx gangs), I found four positive mentors in science and in math. Then in college, I found several more inspiring teachers who supported my interest in research. This continued through graduate school, where I attracted important mentors both inside and outside of UC Berkeley, where I did my graduate work. These intellectual guides included Donald Wilson, Nikolas Tinbergen, Ernst Gellhorn, Hans Selye, and Raymond Dart, all of whom took me under their wings. Subsequently, throughout my development as a body/mind therapist, I was enriched by the grace of more giving, caring, and challenging teachers and therapists, including Ida Rolf and Charlotte Selvers. And now, I find the roles have been reversed, as I am the mentor to hundreds of students. They are in turn guides to their students, who extend their healing influence to thousands of others.

Thank you, Mrs. Kurtz. Thank you for your warmth, your humor, your joy, and your excitement about the world of learning, and for providing a vital episodic memory that drew me to my mentors and them to me. I am convinced that your gentle, friendly touch on my right shoulder over sixty years ago helped change the direction of my life; in fact, I believe it transformed it in ways that I now contemplate with wonder and gratitude. In this very manner, episodic memories can play an important role in creating positive futures. With each subsequent recollection, the memory becomes enriched, making it ever more meaningful. This natural updating is how memories are meant to operate and how they exert their enlivening functions, often just under the threshold of conscious awareness.

Episodic memory helps us to orient in time and space, culling from the past and projecting advantageous outcomes into the future. Most of what we know about this kind of memory comes, of course, from the verbal reports of humans, like mine of Mrs. Kurtz. However, even the "lowly" jaybird exhibits strong evidence of episodic-like memory. Clayton and Dickinson, in their work with the Western scrub jay,[10] were able to demonstrate that these birds possess an episodic-like memory system, one offering a robust survival advantage. This avian species was clearly not only able to remember where they had stashed different food types, but they could recover them discriminately. These recalled distinctions depended on the perishability of the item and the time that had elapsed since hiding it. They were able to remember the "what, where, and when" of specific past caching events and were able to draw from and utilize this information at a later time. Such observed actions, according to these and other researchers, meet the clear behavioral criteria for episodic memory. A similar study was carried out on hummingbirds, demonstrating that they were able to recall where certain flowers were located and how recently these sites were visited. In this way they were able to efficiently maximize fresh nectar targets. Other studies have also demonstrated this same type of episodic-like memory in several different species, including rats, honey bees, dolphins, elephants, and of course, various primates.[11] Like so many of the behaviors we think of as being purely human, episodic memory turns out to have widespread evolutionary taproots. This kind of recollection is not just available for the musings of poets or by the likes of me, in an appreciation of my fifth-grade teacher.

It is generally believed that our earliest episodic memories extend back to the age of three-and-a-half, when the hippocampus becomes significantly functional. However, there is evidence that they can, in some cases, reach back to even earlier ages. Using my mother's corroboration, I can safely say that my earliest episodic memory is from when I was about two-and-a-half years old, sitting by a window near my toddler bed, transfixed by a shaft of light penetrating the still quiet of the room. Dancing dust particles sparkled in the translucent beam. I recall my mother suddenly opening the door and interrupting my dreamy fascination with the scintillating light shaft.* Of course, I didn't know what particles of dust, a light shaft, or scintillation were. It was only much later that I would learn those words and their discriminating definitions. However, that enchanted feeling of sunlit reverie still has a "magical," animating quality that enlivens me to this day. It is the ongoing richness of that mystical memory that encourages me to linger in the present moment and in the spaciousness of light and quiet. It continues to inform my spiritual journey and is updated with every similar, and synchronous, encounter with my deep inner "Self."

Implicit Memory: Emotional and Procedural

Differing radically from both the "cold" declarative and the "warm" episodic memories, implicit memories are "hot" and powerfully compelling. In contrast to the conscious explicit memories (including both declarative and episodic recollections) is the broad category of *implicit memories*. These memories cannot be called up deliberately or accessed as "dreamy" reminiscences. Instead, they arise as a collage of sensations, emotions, and behaviors. Implicit memories appear and disappear surreptitiously, usually far outside the bounds of our conscious awareness. They are primarily organized around emotions and/or skills, or "procedures"—things that the body does automatically (sometimes called "action patterns").

---

* This was verified by my mother. She recalls it well because it was the age I was when we had just moved to a new apartment and I had my own room. Indeed, she remembers seeing me transfixed by the shaft of light.

Even though, in reality, emotional and procedural memories comingle, I will first separate these two types of implicit memories for the purpose of clarification. While emotional memories most certainly have a powerful effect on our behaviors, procedural memories frequently have an even deeper influence—for better or worse—in shaping the trajectory of our lives.

Emotional Rudders

Emotions, according to Darwin's extensive observations, are universal instincts shared by all mammals, a club to which we belong (although we don't always admit to this affiliation) and from which we derive similar instincts. These "mammal-universal" emotions include surprise, fear, anger, disgust, sadness, and joy. I would like to humbly suggest including curiosity, excitement, gladness, and triumph in this collection of innate ("felt-sense") emotions.

The function of emotional memory is to flag and encode important experiences for immediate and potent reference later on. Like bookmarks, emotions are charged signals that select a particular procedural memory out of a book of possible motor memories. They prompt organizing themes for action. In this way, emotional memories interface, well below the level of conscious awareness, with procedural ("body") memories. (See Figure 2.2, insert following page 26.) Emotions provide both relevant survival- and social-based data to inform appropriate responses in any given situation, especially where trying to figure it out mentally would be far too slow and likely off the mark. As such, these memories are vitally important to our individual well-being and that of species survival. It is crucial to appreciate that emotional memories are experienced in the body as physical sensations. Indeed, we see in figure 2.3 clear somatic patterns for each of the primary emotions (insert following page 26).

Emotional memories are generally triggered by features of a present situation in which there are similar types and intensities of emotions. These emotions had, in the past, evoked procedural memories, i.e. survival-based actions (fixed action patterns). While such action responses are often successful strategies, in the case of trauma, they were decidedly and tragically unsuccessful. Such mal-adaptive, habitual reactions leave the individual entangled in unresolved emotional angst, disembodiment, and confusion. However, let's first get a glimpse of the central role played by positive emotions in our shared social humanity.

How Do You Know What I Know about What I Know about You ...

If your everyday practice is to open to your emotions, to all the people you meet, to all the situations you encounter, without closing down, trusting that you can do that—then that will take you as far as you can go. And then you'll understand all the teachings that anyone has ever taught.
—PEMA CHÖDRÖN, BUDDHIST TEACHER

Starting well before Darwin, and extending to the present, countless arrays of theories on emotion have been generated, promoted, abandoned, and eventually discarded. These schemas encompass philosophical, biological, developmental, psychological, and sociological hypotheses. Simply put, however, socially based emotions serve two primary purposes: The first is to signal to others what we are feeling and needing, and the second is to signal to ourselves what we are feeling and needing. This dual function allows two individuals to co-participate in each other's feelings. It is an intimate sharing of internal worlds that is sometimes referred to as "inter-subjectivity."

This type of emotional "resonance" lets me know what you are feeling as well as what I am feeling. We share this connection because our facial and postural expressions of these emotions signal these states to others—but also because the patterned feedback to our brain from receptors in our activated facial and postural muscles (along with feedback from our autonomic nervous system) provides us with the inner feeling of those expressions.

As higher-order functions, emotions let us share what we are feeling about each other, sensing each other's needs and guiding our interactive engagement. From a baby's first cries and smiles to a toddler's trumpeted exhilarations and temper tantrums, from an adolescent's flirtations to an adult's intimate conversations, emotions are a concise form of relational exchange, a primal knowing. Hence, the central role of social emotions is to facilitate our relationship to ourselves and to others. It is also the way we cooperate and how we convey social norms.

Emotions have the potential to connect us to deep parts of ourselves; they are part of the inner prompting that tells us what we need. They are the basis of how we relate to ourselves and get to know ourselves. They are an important part of the connection to our inner knowing, our inner voice, our intuition—to who we really are. Emotions connect us to the very core of how we experience ourselves, with our aliveness, vitality, and purposeful direction in life. Indeed, one of the most vexing "psychological" conditions is *alexithymia,* the inability to connect with, name, and communicate our emotions. This troubling condition is often associated with trauma,[12] and it leaves its sufferers in a state of demoralizing numbness, as if they were "the walking dead."

Let us next turn our attention to the deepest strata of memory, the embedded layer of procedural memories.

PROCEDURAL MEMORY

What the mind has forgotten, the body has not ... thankfully.
—SIGMUND FREUD

While emotional memories are "flags," procedural memories are the impulses, movements, and internal body sensations that guide us through the *how to* of our various actions, skills, attractions, and repulsions. *Procedural memories* can be divided into three broad categories. The first involves *learned motor actions*. These include but are not limited to skills like dancing, skiing, bike riding, and lovemaking. With practice, these "action patterns" can be continuously modified by higher brain regions, as in learning and synchronizing new tango steps and refining sex by incorporating more sensuality and containment, as taught in various Tantric lovemaking practices.

A second category of procedural memory has to do with hardwired *emergency responses* that call upon our basic survival instincts in the face of a threat. These fixed action patterns include bracing, contracting, retracting, fighting, fleeing, and freezing, as well as the setting and maintenance of territorial boundaries. These compelling instinctual emergency responses play a crucial role in the formation and resolution of traumatic memories.*

---

* Although not historically classified as procedural memory, broad clinical experience reinforces the idea that emergency-based survival action patterns can be viewed in this category. Indeed, these fixed action patterns (FAP) are modifiable by selective inhibition from higher (medial) frontal areas so that they exhibit learning features characteristic of other procedural memories.

The third category of procedural memories is the fundamental organismic* response tendencies of *approach or avoidance*, of *attraction or repulsion*. We physically approach that which is likely to be a source of nourishment and growth and avoid sources of injury and toxicity. These avoidance mechanisms include the motor acts of stiffening, retracting, and contracting. On the other hand, those mechanisms of approach involve expanding, extending, and reaching. Patterns of attraction include reaching for a person close to us or moving toward things we want in our lives. Those patterns of avoidance include steering clear of foods that don't smell or taste right, or avoiding individuals who seem "emotionally toxic" to us.

These movement patterns, of approach and avoidance, form the underlying primitive motivational rudders in our lives. They are the action blueprints of all living organisms, from those of the lowly amoeba to our complex humanoid interactions with the world and each other. In this way they are a compass that guides us through life. We can think of these basic functions (sometimes called "hedonic valences") as a traffic light with yellow (alert and assess), green (approach), and red (avoid). What follows is an example of the often hidden motivations of these internal cues and how we use them to navigate around obstacles and toward nourishment.

Arnold and Me

Please bear with me as I offer another personal example. The following vignette illustrates the enlivening weave of procedural, emotional, episodic, and declarative memory functions in the fabric of our lives.

---

* An organism is defined as a complex living system having properties and functions determined not only by the properties and relations of its individual parts, but also by the character of the whole that they compose and by the relations of the parts to the whole.

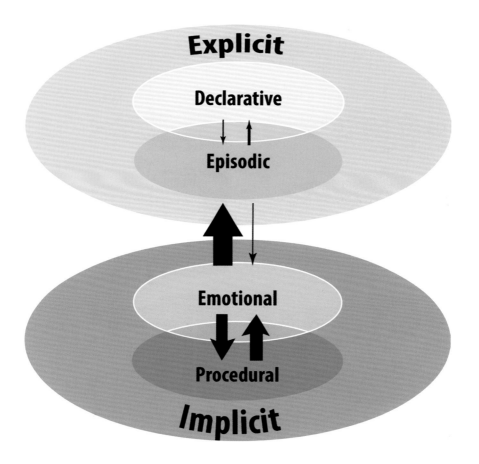

Figure 2.2 Interrelationship between Memory Systems

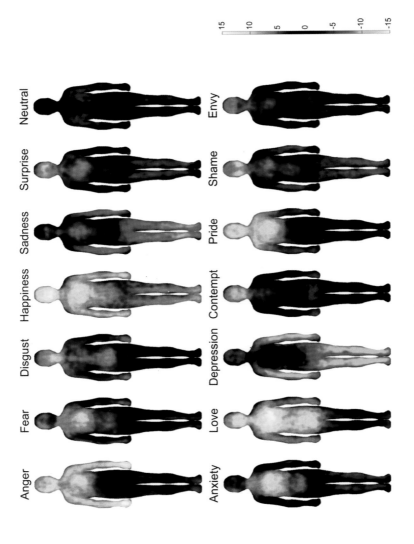

Figure 2.3 Emotional Bodily Signatures (Source: Lauri Nummenmaa, Enrico Glerean, Riitta Hari, and Jari. K. Hietanen, "Bodily Maps of Emotions," *Proceedings of the National Academy of Sciences* 111, no. 2 (January 2014): 646–651, http://www.pnas.org/cgi/doi/10.1073/pnas.1321664111.)

About twenty-five years ago I was visiting my parents in New York City. After a day of museum hopping, I took the uptown D train. It was rush hour and the car was densely packed with family men in various shades of gray, most with newspapers folded neatly under their arms. One particularly tall man caught my attention. As I glanced at him, I experienced a vague visceral feeling of warmth and an uncanny sense of being at ease with this stranger. I experienced this as a particular expansion or spaciousness in my chest and belly, coupled with a faint desire to approach him. Both of us departed the train at 205th street, the last stop in the Bronx. I followed a peculiar impulse in my legs to walk up to him and found myself touching his arm. We gazed at each other with shared curiosity. The name "Arnold" fell unexpectedly from my lips. I don't know who was more surprised as we stood, perplexed, looking at each other for some moments. It was then that I realized that Arnold and I were classmates in the first grade—some forty years before this chance encounter on the train.

At six years old I was by far the smallest child in the class. I had disproportionately large ears and was frequently bullied. Arnold was the one kid who had consistently befriended me. In this way, we had laid the foundation for an enduring emotional relationship. The stored imprint of his kind protection remained dormant in my emotional and procedural memory banks for decades; that is, until the momentary postural and facial recognition cues led me to approach him and discover the emerging context of our shared history.

As I walked up the hill to my parents' apartment I felt my spine lengthen, as though lifted by an invisible string gently coaxing my head skyward. There was a notable bounce in my step. I was moved by a stream of images and feelings from the first grade. Along with these episodic memories and accompanying sensations of spaciousness in my chest, I was able to reflect on some moments of distress.

I remembered how my classmates taunted me with the nickname "Dumbo" (as in the Disney elephant) because of my large ears.

Then, just as I entered the apartment building, I felt a clear physical sensation of strength in my legs and arms, and a swelling pride in my chest. With that procedural awareness, another episodic memory then materialized, recalling the last time I was attacked, some sixty-plus years ago. I had been cornered by two of the cruelest bullies—twins, in fact. I could still see their mean, mocking faces as they forced me out onto Gun Hill Road and into the rush of oncoming traffic. To all of our amazement, I started to swing wildly with my arms, moving defiantly toward them. They stopped dead in their tracks. Their expressions flipped dramatically, from ridicule and scorn to startle and fear, as they ran away. That was the last time I was bullied. After that I was treated with respect and invited to play games with the other kids.

This episode illustrates the enduring importance of procedural and emotional memories as embodied resources that are available to be drawn upon throughout our lives. When I first registered Arnold on the train, my emerging "memory" was a faint *implicit* one—a strange fascination with him that was utterly devoid of content or context. This procedural memory played out as a lingering gaze, a slight expansion of my chest, an extension of my spine, and then a warm, spacious feeling in my belly. However, as I approached him, and as his name fell from my lips, I was beginning to transition from an implicit, procedural memory (body sensations, postures, motor impulses) to an emotional memory (surprise, curiosity), and then to an episodic memory that I could drift with and reflect upon. (See Figure 2.2, insert following page 26.)

With the door to the past cracked opened, I could more consciously recall snippets, or episodic memories, of that year-long saga: joining the class midway through the year because of my age; registering the discomfort of feeling out of place; sensing how Arnold had supported me to gain my own strength and confidence as a child; and finally reconnecting to how I had triumphed by standing up to the class bullies and gaining the acceptance of the other children. In the midst of these episodic memories, I could feel the readiness and power in my arms and shoulders as I imagined myself striking out against the bullies. It was in this moment that my episodic memory once again evoked the procedural ones of defense, strength, and self-protection. Walking boldly and energetically up the stairs to the apartment, I felt warm, grateful, and proud. I could now describe this episodic memory as a coherent story in a declarative, narrative form.

Compared to my initial procedural attraction to Arnold on the train, the remembrances of my first-grade encounters, as episodic memories, were recalled as I walked to my parents' building. These were reviewed at a relatively conscious level even though they were primarily spontaneous. Like the madeleine in Proust's *Remembrances of Things Past,* my uncanny (procedural) attraction to Arnold was evoked by an *implicit trigger.* In Proust's case, this trigger was the taste of a tea-dipped pastry. He did not think, "Oh, this pastry reminds me of the time, as a child, when my mother would give me a cup of tea with a madeleine, and that reminded me of my walk to school." Rather, the *sensorial experience* of tea plus a madeleine triggered procedural, episodic, and emotional processes that were largely subconscious. For me, the trigger was the remote and implicit recognition of the manifold shapes and contours of Arnold's face, his posture, and his movements. Without conscious awareness, I somehow sorted through the hundreds of thousands of faces, bodies, postures, and gaits that I had been exposed to in the course of my life and then extrapolated these patterns from childhood to a forty-six-year-old man! The only reason this was possible was that Arnold—nearly forty years before—had a powerful physical, emotional, and relational effect on me.

If as adults we happen to encounter a childhood acquaintance on the street, there is a good likelihood that we will not consciously recognize them. However, we might well experience a particular feeling tone and relational context: happiness, if they befriended us, or fear, if they bullied us. In other words, we might differentiate between friend and foe, yet have no idea of their names, or from where we might have known them, or even that we ever did know them—that is, until the emotional procedural memory transitions into an episodic collage and then into a declarative form. A supercomputer, like IBM's Watson, would be thoroughly challenged to perform such a complex pattern-recognition task. Even the most sophisticated supercomputers, and their elite programmers, are unable to recognize and utilize "emotional tones" the way humans and animals do. This is the manifest power of implicit memories in registering emotionally nuanced, relational experiences and continuously computing meanings throughout the developmental arc of our life.

The capacity to move between implicit and explicit memory, from less conscious to more conscious (and vice-versa), is also an important theme in integrating traumatic experiences and in generally learning about who we were, who we are, and who we are becoming. My memory of Arnold demonstrates the value of this coherent communication between implicit and explicit memory systems. It is the fluid relationship between sensation, feeling, image, and action that allowed me to weave a fresh new adult narrative, one that enhanced my sense of mastery, triumph, vitality, and selfhood. For me, this renewed confidence and sense of my own strength and agency was timely. I believe it helped provide a foundation to fortify my resolve to relinquish an energy-draining "day job" and take hold of the freedom needed to unleash my creativity. It perhaps even gave me the confidence to devote all of my efforts to financially supporting myself outside of the halls of academia and industry. This independent agency energized my pursuit of the therapeutic vision that became Somatic Experiencing, my life's work. Indeed, this journey illustrates the importance of procedural memories as deeply *embodied resources* in the forward movement of our lives.

How many people like Arnold "live" inside our psyches, enhancing or haunting our emotions and controlling our bodily reactions? Though we may be little aware of their existence, we are nonetheless under their shadow, for better or worse. Indeed, these implicit memories are generally activated below the radar of our conscious awareness, often when we least expect or desire them to show up. To break these negative "complexes" (often associated with our parents) and enhance positive ones, we need to develop a capacity for self-exploration and reflective self-awareness. My story about Arnold is an example of how we can open to this curiosity and exploration about our lives and how it can enliven and empower us.

The crucial importance of emotions, procedures, and narratives in making sense of our world is also illustrated in the following case study, in which this critical integrative weaving of implicit and explicit memory has completely broken down. David is a neurological patient whose behaviors demonstrate what happens when the various memory systems are inaccessible to each other—when they are absent, disconnected, or disassociated, as they are to some degree in the case of trauma.

David, Marooned on an Island

David, suffering from severe brain damage to his limbic system, has lived in a group home for the mentally disabled most of his adult life. The caretakers at the institution began to note an interesting quirk in David's behaviors: Still retaining his taste for food and other sensory fulfillments, he would often make requests of the other patients for cigarettes or morsels of food. The staff noticed that he always seemed to gravitate toward certain residents, and his requests of these specific people seemed to become progressively more frequent. In a chance observation, David's body was noted to startle, jerk, and "freeze" when he happened to encounter a particular unfriendly person while walking in the corridor. He would then abruptly turn away and walk on as if nothing had happened.

If we were merely to observe David's everyday behaviors, he would appear to be quite normal. We would see him move toward people who in the past had been helpful to him and avoid those who had not. It would seem that he had an intact capacity to discern people's intentions and to respond appropriately. However, in spite of his seeming capacity to recognize different patients by repeatedly approaching or avoiding them, just moments later, he would be unable to remember with whom he had just had the interaction or to consciously recognize their face. But, apparently *his body did remember,* because he seemed to vary his approach or avoidance to a specific person, somehow retaining the outcome of each previous encounter.

All kinds of intellectual tests showed that David's intelligence was above average. No purely cognitive reasoning tests could be devised that would indicate any intellectual deficits—quite the opposite. In fact, his ability to reason intellectually, when it did *not* involve an emotional or relational association, was fully retained. In this regard David appeared completely normal, perhaps unusually clever, and of high IQ. More sophisticated tests, however, showed that David's capacity to make moral judgments (which require subtle emotional and relational tones) was profoundly impaired.

Antonio Damasio, the well-known consulting neurologist at the home, devised a clever "good cop, bad cop" experiment designed to assess David's behaviors and brain function.[13] Damasio asked different members of the staff to behave in a consistent manner whenever David approached them. One group responded only with a friendly smile and was always helpful to him. Members of the second group were unfriendly and said things to confuse him. A third group remained neutral to his advances.

David was then asked to participate in a photographic "lineup." In viewing four photos—one friendly individual, one unfriendly, one neutral, and one photograph of someone he had never seen before—he was completely unable to name or select the person with whom he just had the interaction. It was as though these people didn't exist to him. However, in spite of this glaring incapacity for conscious facial identification (as evidenced by the lineup) in an actual social situation, his body moved toward, and he selectively chose, the person who was friendly, while obviously avoiding the unfriendly stooges. This selection reoccurred *over 80 percent of the time*. Furthermore, one person who was selected to be an unfriendly figure in the experiment was a young, beautiful, and naturally warm female research assistant. David, who had the reputation of being quite the flirt with a strong attraction to pretty women, rarely approached her for his requests. Eighty percent of the time he chose the average-looking man who was consistently friendly to him.

What was it that allowed David to choose certain people when he was (consciously) unable to even recognize any of their faces or identify them by name? Clearly, he had an intact *procedural* memory of previous encounters with these individuals. This record was displayed by his definitive approach or avoidance behaviors—*his body visibly remembered*, even though "he" had no conscious memory of the encounters. In choosing kindness and avoiding frosty rejection, his body was in some way directed by certain (implicit) sensate procedures, those valences of *approach versus avoidance*.

As a result of the severe brain injury to his temporal lobes, David had lost the function of the middle parts of his brain, the areas where we register emotions and relationships. His injury had obliterated a significant portion of his temporal lobes, including the amygdala and hippocampus, two structures involved with emotion and short-term (spatial-temporal) memory and learning. This specific affliction left David marooned, alone on an island, separated from his past and future, and unable to make moral judgments and form relationships that extended beyond the immediate present. It was a nightmarish scenario of which he apparently remained "fortunately" unaware.

In spite of all of his impairments, David was somehow able to calculate and execute a complex behavioral approach-versus-avoidance decision that he was not at all consciously aware of. Because of his intact ability to selectively approach or avoid, we can presume these "decisions" must have taken place in the upper brain stem, including the thalamus, cerebellum, and the involuntary extrapyramidal motor system. These procedures and "proto-emotions" were calculated *below* the level of the emotional brain (which no longer existed due to his severe injury) and completely out of reach of his (reasoning) neocortex. This unconscious, upper–brain stem determination of approach versus avoidance was even strong enough to override his "lewd" impulses toward the pretty, but unpleasant, female stooge.

It is highly unlikely that David's decision to approach a particular friendly staff member transpired in his (fully functioning) cerebral cortex. Normally, when we see a face, many of us might naively assume that we first analyze it in our mind and then, based on our conscious observations, *think* and assess whether this person might be friendly or unfriendly—and then respond appropriately. If David's discernment of a friendly versus unfriendly person and his "decision" to approach rather than avoid them had occurred in the conscious neocortex, he would have then had a reliable declarative memory of his encounters and would surely have been able to pick the correct person in Damasio's lineup. Clearly this was not the case.

David's decision to approach or to avoid the stooges could not have occurred in his emotional (temporal-limbic) brain region either, as this entire area was inoperative due to extensive damage. So the only remaining part of his brain that could be making these complex "decisions" would be the region of his brain stem, cerebellum, and thalamus. However, without the intermediary of the limbic brain (responsible for emotions and relationships), he was unable to "upload" information from the primitive brain stem (body-based valences of approach versus avoidance) to the limbic brain, where it would have registered the felt quality and context of his relationship with the stooges. Here, the information would have been stored as an emotional memory. Then, in turn, this limbic (emotional) memory would normally be uploaded to the frontal cerebral cortex, where it would then be recorded, accessed, and compiled as episodic and declarative memories that contained names and faces. In David, however, this sequential processing was completely lacking and couldn't reach the cerebral cortex, not because of an insufficiency in the cortex (which was not damaged, as evidenced by his well-above-average IQ), but because he was unable to record emotional memories based upon his (accurate) brain stem procedural valences of approach or avoidance.

The only reasonable conclusion that can be made here is that there exists, in the upper brain stem and thalamus, a complex assessment-making capacity, one that consistently allows for an undeniable—80 percent—accuracy and a highly differentiated decision tree for making implicit choices between approach (nourishment) and avoidance (threat). Such apparent decision making, at the brain stem level, flies in the face of what is generally accepted about human memory and consciousness.

Central to the theme of this book is that the existence of procedural memories, which lie well below normal waking consciousness, is a key in clinically working with traumatic memories.

4

EMOTIONS, PROCEDURAL MEMORIES, AND THE STRUCTURE OF TRAUMA

This chapter begins with a discussion of how procedural memories form the bedrock of our sensations, as well as many of our feelings, thoughts, and beliefs. In addition, we will discuss how procedural memories can be accessed to "renegotiate" a trauma, whether it is a debilitating, "large-T" Trauma or a seemingly inconsequential, "small-t" trauma.

You'll recall from Chapter 3 that the critically important subcategory of implicit memories, called *procedural* memories, involves movement patterns. These *action programs* include: 1) learned motor skills, 2) valences of approach/avoidance,[14] and 3) survival reactions. The latter two engage *innate movement programs* (action patterns), which are charged by evolution to carry out actions that are necessary for our survival and well-being.

It is the persistence, power, and longevity of procedural memories that make them critical when considering any therapeutic protocol. It is important to note that of all the memory subsystems, those of the instinctual survival reactions are the deepest, most compelling, and, in times of threat and stress, generally override the other implicit and explicit memory subtypes. (See Figure 4.1, insert following page 42.)

Let us first consider an example of a procedural memory as an *acquired motor skill*. Learning to ride a bicycle may seem like a formidable, if not terrifying, task, yet with the gentle support of a parent or older sibling, we master the quixotic forces of gravity, velocity, and momentum. We do this *procedurally*, without any explicit knowledge of the physics or math involved. We learn to master these forces largely by trial and error; the requisite learning curve is, of necessity, quite steep. The adage that one never forgets how to ride a bike rings true for most procedural memories, for better or for worse. So if during one of our early bicycling efforts we have the misfortune of hitting loose gravel and taking a nasty spill, the acquisition of adaptive and requisite balanced movements and body postures can be interfered with. Then when we finally do ride, it may be with a hesitancy leading to instability, or, alternatively, with daredevil abandon and "counter phobia." What should have evolved into a nuanced learned motor skill is overridden and becomes instead a habitual, survival-based reactive pattern of bracing and contracting, or of overcompensating with counter-phobic risk taking; both are less-than-optimal outcomes and unfortunate examples of the durability of a procedural memory. *Indeed, persistent maladaptive procedural and emotional memories form the core mechanism that underlies all traumas, as well as many problematic social and relationship issues.*

Over time, through trial and error, success and failure, our bodies gather which movement strategies work and which ones don't. For example, which situations should we approach and from which should we retreat? In which should we engage with "fight or flight," and when should we "freeze" and remain motionless? A specific example of the persistence of maladaptive procedural memories (involving approach/avoidance and survival reactions) is manifested in Ana, who was raped as a child by her grandfather and now as an adult stiffens, retracts, and finally collapses in fear and revulsion when caressed by her loving husband. Her demoralizing confusion between a safe and a dangerous person is compounded by a sur-vival-based bias to assume danger even where there exists only the most superficial of similarities—in this case, the combined triggers of men and touch. Therefore, Ana's trauma—whether consciously remembered or not—compels the unfortunate mistake of perceiving a threat of violation by her dearest, most caring friend.

In Ana's therapy she allows herself to feel a physical impulse to pull away from her husband, suggesting an incomplete survival-based reaction. This resides as a procedural memory, devoid of con-tent, yet playing out as if she were in the clutches of her grandfather. Sensing more deeply how her body stiffens and contracts gives rise to a spontaneous image of the grandfather and the smell of his cigarette-laden breath. Ana then experiences an urge to push him off. Upon focusing on that impulse, she feels a tentative power in her arms along with the self-compassionate realization that she couldn't have pushed him off as a child. She then feels a surge of anger and a sustained strength as she pushes (the image of) him away. Ana then feels a wave of nausea as her forehead breaks out in beads of sweat. This autonomic reaction satisfies and completes the drive to repel her grandfather; it is an important part of the reworking of the original thwarted response to the procedural memory of trying to get away from him. This auto-nomic reaction is followed by a full deep breath, a spreading warmth in her hands, and then an unexpected calm. Ana notes with gratitude that she is now looking forward to returning home. At her next visit she reports that she was able to enjoy her husband's touch and felt secure in his arms. She requests that we now work toward gradually prepar-ing her for some initial sexual exploration with her cherished husband.

Friend or Foe?

As introduced in Chapter 3, mild emotions and nuanced feelings serve the dynamic function of forming and sustaining relationships in times of relative safety. They do this by communicating important social information to others, as well as to ourselves. These ambient emotional feelings fulfill the function of *guiding* us in social situations and generating intragroup cohesion. They accomplish this via a wide range of feelings, particularly those that we know to be positive or "eudemonic," such as joy, caring, belonging, purposefulness, cooperation, and peacefulness. When we encounter a friend whom we have not seen for a while, we are filled with joy and gladness. Or if someone dear to us leaves or passes on, we may first grieve and then be filled with a cleansing sadness and fond remembrances.*

Sometimes, low to moderate levels of anger alert us when something is interfering with a relationship or a task. Then, hopefully, that anger guides, motivates, and empowers us to remove the obstacle, thus restoring the relationship and moving forward. At moderate levels, emotions may signal the *possibility* of danger. We convey this potentiality to others through body language, via our postures and facial expressions. As social animals, when sensing danger in the environment, we stiffen in readiness, preparing ourselves for action while alerting others, and then can cooperatively take protective, evasive, defensive, or aggressive action.

Intense levels of fear, anger, terror, or rage compel us to instantaneously and unequivocally act with full-out power in action by unconsciously selecting and evoking specific procedural memories for fighting or fleeing. If we cannot fully execute these actions or are overwhelmed, we freeze or collapse in helpless immobility, conserving our energy until safety is restored. In summary, when high levels of activation surge forth and intense emotions take over, they can "flip" us into the procedural survival programs of "kill

---

* The Brazilians have a name for this tender feeling: *saudade*. The definition of this word includes feeling the loss of someone dear to you, but still holding them in your heart such that they are never really gone, but with you eternally.

or be killed" (fight-or-flight) mode, or de-enervate us into collapse, shame, defeat, and helplessness.

Generally, moderate to high levels of subcortically evoked intense "negative" emotions, particularly those of fear and anger, cue us to danger and prompt us to locate its source, evaluate its actual threat, and then call forth the actions necessary to defend or protect ourselves and others. However, this option for action will be (appropriately) moot if our assessment yields an absence of danger. In this case we ideally return to a fluid state of *relaxed alertness.*

Who among us hasn't experienced a moment of inexplicable fear and stiffening when startled by a novel sound or shifting shadow, yet only a few seconds later easily identified the potential "danger" and assessed its actual salience and risk? More often than not, this charged, attention-grabbing, emotionally tagged event is something benign, like a door opening abruptly or a curtain billowing in the wind. If we have a balanced, resilient nervous system our "here and now" observing-ego/prefrontal cortex says to the emotionally charged amygdala, "Chill out. Relax. It's just a door being opened by your friend John, who has arrived early for our meeting." *Hence, when we are able to stand back, observe, and reduce the intensity of these emotions, we are afforded the possibility of also selecting and modifying the survival responses themselves.*

In an intriguing incidence of synchronicity, while working on this very chapter, Laura (my editor) and I needed a stretch break, so we took a leisurely walk by the lake at Mythenquai, one of the many beautiful parks in Zurich. We were meandering among the children splashing in the shallow wading pools and playing on the swings and jungle gyms, relaxing in the soft, sun-filled warmth and opening to the gentle wonders of the day, taking pleasure in our sensory-rich environment. Then, almost in unison, we found ourselves stopping, startled, and momentarily breathless. Simultaneously, we scanned our surroundings, zeroing in on a thicket of tall bamboo.

Taking quick notice of several twenty-foot stalks that were inexplicably bending and shaking, we stood alert, tensed and hyper-focused, seeking to identify the source of threat and readying to exit posthaste. Nothing but the movement of the bamboo occupied our awareness. The aperture of our sensory field constricted abruptly, and the luxurious pleasures of the park all but vanished.

For our distant ancestors in dense jungles, this pattern of movement and rustling could have easily signaled a stalking, crouching tiger. However, this time-honed instinctual reaction was patently ridiculous given that this was the least likely place on earth to encounter a threat of any kind! Indeed, on a second look, we realized it was just a group of errant children, not obeying the tidy norms of the Swiss, but instead hiding in the dense bamboo, playing Tarzan of the jungle. They were gleefully forcing some of the tallest stalks to bend steeply; obviously no cause for alarm, just a chuckle. Such an exaggerated, fear-cued reaction to a maximally benign situation is an example of what is technically called a *false-positive*. Initially, we reacted "positively" as though the shaking bamboo were a real threat, even though (in this case) it turned out to be just a "false alarm"—a false-positive.

False-Positive Bias

In nature, as in the park in Zurich, the consequence of a false-positive assessment is relatively minor. Really, nothing was lost, other than the expenditure of a few extra calories, when we mistook the mischievous children for a mythical tiger in Mythenquai Park. On the other hand, *false-negatives*—acting as though something is not dangerous when in fact it actually is—can be fatal and are evolutionarily unsustainable. If we ignore the rustling in the bushes, we may become easy prey for a stalking mountain lion or a hungry bear. Hence, it is better that any uncertainty or ambiguity is experienced as a threat (i.e., that we have a strong innate bias toward false-positives) and then later, after

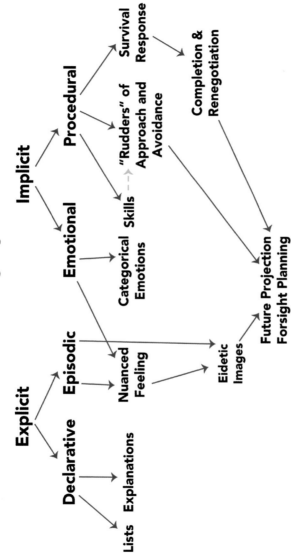

Figure 4.1 Relationships between explicit and implicit memory systems in planning and future projection (moving forward in life).

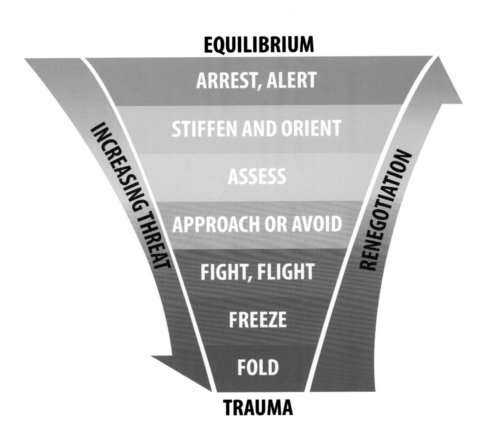

Figure 4.2 Escalating levels of threat (left side) lead to traumatic states. We "renegotiate" threat by moving upwards from trauma toward alertness, orientation, and equilibrium (right side).

the initial startle, correctly identified as safe; nothing gained, nothing lost. So when, rather than a stalking predator, we discover the source of a startling noise to be playing children or a flock of birds taking flight, it is still better from an evolutionary vantage point to have first automatically presumed it to be a lethal threat. In other words, always give the benefit of the doubt to the worst-case scenario.* Our abrupt and escalating emotions of startle and fear instruct us to immediately take heed.

However, when these intense emotions and their attendant motor responses (procedural memories) become chronic, the very emotions that are intended to serve, guide, protect, and defend us can become corrosive and turn against us—against the Self. It is critical at this point to understand how to work with these maladaptive emotions and procedural engrams. "Renegotiation" is a means of resolving these traumatic memories through the gentle release of chronic emotions and the creative restructuring of the dysfunctional responses. This provides us with an avenue of return to our pre-trauma capacity for balance and well-being.

Renegotiation

Renegotiation is not about simply reliving a traumatic experience. It is, rather, the gradual and titrated *revisiting* of various sensory-motor elements comprising a particular trauma engram. Renegotiation occurs primarily by accessing procedural memories associated with the two dysregulated states of the autonomic nervous

---

* Any new meditator observes this innate bias as they try to deflect the intrusive deluge of obsessive worry and negative thoughts, hopefully stilling the voracious "monkey mind" with the guidance of a compassionate and experienced teacher. It is our evolutionary bias toward a false-positive that can seriously interfere with the capacity to meditate as it prompts the mind to, habitually, wander toward fear and worry.

system (ANS)—hyperarousal/overwhelm or hypoarousal/shutdown and helplessness—and then restoring and completing the associated active responses. As this process progresses, the client moves from hypo- or hyperarousal, toward equilibrium, relaxed alertness, and a here-and-now orientation. (See Figure 4.2, insert following page 42 and Figure 5.2, insert following page 58.) In essence, renegotiation as a therapeutic process reverses the sequence of the biological action in response to threat. Finally, to complete the therapeutic process, the renegotiated procedural memories are linked to the recalibrated episodic and narrative memories.

In review, emotional arousal in response to threat exists on a continuum, but with abrupt amplifications at certain points within that spectrum. These emotions are signals that evoke innate (pre-pared) motor action programs. This continuum begins with mild arousal (curiosity) in response to novelty in the environment and moves smoothly through to pleasure/displeasure until the abrupt shift into fear, rage, terror, and horror. The sequence of evoked motor patterns and their associated emotions is as follows:

1. Arrest and alert—associated with curiosity.
2. Stiffen and orient—associated with focused attention, inter-est, and preparedness.
3. Assess—associated with intense interest, friendliness, or repulsion. This assessment is informed by our genetic mem-ory banks, as well as our personal histories.
4. Approach or avoid—associated with pleasure and displeasure.

In the more intense activation states, there is an abrupt shift to the powerfully compelling emotions of fear, rage, terror, and horror that erupt into all-out action, immobilization or collapse:

5. Fight-or-flight—experienced as fear. When these active responses are thwarted we:
6. Freeze, as in "scared stiff"—associated with terror.
7. "Fold" and collapse—associated with helpless/hopeless horror.

During our "jungle encounter" at Mythenquai Park, Laura and I went through the first three phases of the above sequence. Once the source of possible threat was identified and readily assessed as nonthreatening, our response was one of shared mirth. Hence, it can be seen that when the experience of likely threat is minimal, these early phases will reverse naturally and readily, returning the organism (in this case, both Laura and me) to a state of relaxed alertness. However, when these initial response phases to potential threat do not sufficiently terminate the alarm, the call to action escalates abruptly. Indeed, if the rustling bamboo had revealed a stalking predator, our emotional state would have intensified dramatically and mobilized our full-out action responses in a life-or-death, biologically ordained survival sequence (Phases 5, 6, and 7).

In general, the emergency-based emotions in Phases 5, 6, and 7 evoke an intensifying sequence of procedural motor programs that increase along a gradient, from a sense of danger in fight-or-flight, to acute fear in freeze, and then finally to the helpless terror and the "last-ditch" default reaction of collapse and shutdown. These innate procedural responses have distinct autonomic nervous system (ANS) features. Phase 5, fight-or-flight, is supported by the sympathetic-adrenal system, thus mobilizing us to meet the emergency. Then, if the threat is not resolved or our defensive/protective actions are thwarted, Phase 6, freeze, takes over. This is accompanied by an intensification of the already activated sympathetic-adrenal arousal, springing us into hyper-drive and simultaneous immobility; we become "scared stiff." Once the threat level is perceived as inescapable or mortal, we progress to Phase 7, "folding," a profound state of hopelessness and helplessness. Our bodies and spirit collapse while our metabolic processes (including digestion, respiration, circulation, and energy production) shut down. This state of shutdown is mediated by the so-called primitive (unmyelinated) branch of the parasympathetic nervous system via the vagus (tenth cranial) nerve.[15] In this state, with both the accelerator and brake fully engaged, the autonomic dynamics are such that we may flip back and forth almost instantaneously between sympathetic and parasympathetic (vagal) dominance (hyper- and hypoarousal); see Figure 5.2, insert following page 58.[16] When people become "stuck" in this unstable, paroxysmal phase, they are left in the sheer hell realm of trauma, paralyzed with terror, while experiencing eruptions of blind rage yet devoid of the sustained energy to act.

To renegotiate a trauma, the defense-orienting sequence must be reversed by first attending to the completion of the relevant procedural memories of Phases 5, 6, and 7. We do this by resolving these highly activated states and restoring a more active response where there has been shutdown. In doing this, we successively move back up the chain: from 7 to 6 to 5 to 4 to 3 to 2 to 1.* In this sequential renegotiation, the individual will return to a here-and-now orientation, with a deepened regulation and inner balance. This completion is evidenced by a restoration of the ANS into its range of dynamic equilibrium and relaxed alertness. (See Figure 4.2, insert following page 42.)

SIBAM

Therapeutically, renegotiation and transformation are clarified and guided by a map of a person's inner experience. The SIBAM Model incorporates the neurophysiologic, somatic, sensory, behavioral, and affective aspects of an individual's experience, whether traumatic or triumphant. In a nontraumatized state, the elements of SIBAM (sensation, image, behavior, affect, and meaning) form a fluid, continuous, and coherent response that is appropriate to the present situation. In this way, coherent narratives evolve from primitive sensory-motor processing. However, where there is

---

* It should be noted that this sequence is by no means linear, and it frequently takes several passes to renegotiate a trauma.

unresolved trauma, elements of SIBAM are either too closely linked (over-coupled), or dissociated and fragmented (under-coupled). The concept of SIBAM, and its utilization in renegotiating trauma, is described in detail in Chapter 7 of my book *In an Unspoken Voice*.[17]

Sensation

These are the interoceptive, physical sensations that arise from within the body, including (from most conscious to least conscious):

- Kinesthetic—muscle tension patterns
- Proprioceptive—awareness of our position in space
- Vestibular—acceleration and deceleration
- Visceral—sensations from the viscera (guts, heart, and lungs) and blood vessels

Image

Image refers to the external sense impressions, which include sight, taste, smell, hearing, and touch (the tactile sense).

Behavior

Behavior is the only channel that the therapist is able to observe directly. The therapist can infer a client's inner states from reading his or her body's language. These include:

- Voluntary gestures
- Emotional/facial expressions
- Posture—the platforms from which intrinsic movement is initiated; typically refers to the spine.
- Autonomic signals—includes the cardiovascular and respiratory systems. The pulse rate can be measured by the client's carotid artery in the neck.
- Visceral behavior—digestive shifts can be "observed" via changing sounds in the gut.
- Archetypal behaviors—include involuntary gestures or postural shifts that convey a universal meaning.

Affect

Affect refers to the categorical emotions of fear, anger, sadness, joy, and disgust, as well as contours of feelings. Contours are the nuanced, sensation-based (felt sense) feelings of attraction and avoidance, of "goodness" and "badness," that guide us throughout our lives. They are the rudders and bearings that take us through the day.

Meaning

Meanings are the labels we attach to the totality of experience from the combined elements of S, I, B, and A. These include trauma-based fixed beliefs. The therapist helps the client to freely access the full spectrum of developing sensations and feelings to form new meanings, allowing the old cognitive beliefs of "badness" to transform as part of the process of renegotiation.

Using SIBAM: A Case Study

What follows is a simple example of utilizing SIBAM with a client to address her trigger for a relatively minor trauma. Louise loves nature, parks, meadows, and grassy knolls; however, every time she smells newly mown grass she feels nauseated, anxious, and dizzy. Her fixated belief (M) is that she might have an allergy to grass and that it is something to be avoided. The olfactory and visual image (I), the smell and sight of cut grass, is associated with—or (over) coupled to—the sensations of nausea and dizziness (S) coming from her visceral and vestibular systems. She has no idea why this happens; she just knows that she has a strong dislike (M) of cut grass. As Louise explores her sensations and images, seeing and smelling cut grass in her "mind's eye," she takes time to explore her bodily sensations in detail. As she does this, she has an emergent new sensation of being spun in the air while held by her left wrist and left ankle. This experience is both vestibular (S) as well as a feeling of pressure on her wrist and ankle (I). She next gets a tactile and visual image of her bully brother forcefully holding her wrists and giving her an unwelcome and frightening airplane spin on the (freshly cut) front lawn of her childhood home when she was four or five years old. She experiences her body trying to contract into a ball that would break the momentum of the spin (S). As she evokes this active defensive response, she has another impulse (S) to dig the fingernails of her right hand into his flesh. She now feels power in her hands, arms, and chest (S) as she imagines doing this.

Louise feels a momentary fear (A) as she trembles and breathes, yet it quickly subsides as she realizes that she is no longer in danger. She opens her eyes and orients (B) by looking around the colorful office. Then turning her head a bit farther, she greets the open face of her therapist with a quiet smile (B). Feeling intact with this newfound safety, she settles. She then experiences a deep, spontaneous breath (B) and reports feeling secure in her belly now (S), a new visceral awareness. She pauses and then notices some lingering tightness around her wrist (S). She registers an impulse to try and pry her hands loose (S, kinesthetic). Feeling a wave of anger (A) building up inside her, she yells, "Stop!" by using the motor muscles of her vocal cords (B). She settles again and feels the tactile pleasure of lying on the soft, newly mown grass, taking in the warmth of the summertime sunshine (I). Fresh grass is no longer over-coupled with the unpleasant sensations (old M); new green, freshly groomed grass is good, parks are wonderful places, and "all is well" (new M and coherent narrative).

Once we understand the process of renegotiation and engage its transformative power, biology works to move the experience along. It follows naturally that when the client's bodily responses are elaborated and become conscious in the safety of the present moment, the thwarted procedural memories come to an intrinsic corrective experience and there is resolution.

Working in a phased sequence of renegotiation, as we observed in the session with Louise, continually strengthens the *critical observer function.* This is the capacity to stay present and track the various troubling sensations, emotions, and images—to meet them without being overwhelmed. This function, in turn, facilitates coming to peace with one's memory amalgams.

With this basic understanding of renegotiation, we'll study in the next chapter Pedro's trauma transformation and rite of passage, his personal hero's journey, as he masters his disempowered memories, allowing them to evolve from procedural/emotional memory into an episodic narrative.

5

A HERO'S JOURNEY

*Primordial feelings provide a direct experience of one's own
living body, wordless, unadorned, and connected to nothing
but sheer existence. These primordial feelings reflect the current
state of the body along varied dimensions ... along the scale that
ranges from pleasure to pain, and they originate at the level of
the brain stem rather than the cerebral cortex. All feelings of
emotion are complex musical variations on primordial feelings.*
—ANTONIO DAMASIO, THE FEELING OF WHAT HAPPENS

The transformation of procedural memories, from immobility
and helplessness to hyperarousal and mobilization, and finally to
triumph and mastery, is a trajectory I have consistently observed
in most of the thousands of traumatized individuals that I have
worked with over the past forty-five years. Pedro is an example of
this primordial awakening.

Pedro

Pedro is a fifteen-year-old adolescent suffering from Tourette's
syndrome, severe claustrophobia, and panic attacks, as well as
intermittent asthma like symptoms. He was brought to one of my
case consultations during a class I was conducting in Brazil by

his mother, Carla. Pedro was obviously very uncomfortable with the idea of talking to a therapist, particularly in a group setting. However, his desire to get relief from the embarrassment and shame about his "tics" and panic attacks helped him overcome his reluctance to attend the session. His tics involved myoclonic jerks and convulsions in the muscles of his neck and face, causing abrupt lateral movements of the jaw and repetitive turning of the head to the right. In taking a history from his mother, I learned his childhood had included significant, serious falls involving repeated shocks to his head. A brief accounting of these incidents is as follows.

At seven months of age, Pedro tumbled several feet out of his crib and landed facedown on the floor. The child's nanny had discounted the muffled noise of the infant's terrified screams, reassuring his mother that nothing was amiss with her baby. Though not yet crawling, Pedro had managed to scoot himself to the closed bedroom door. Fifteen or twenty minutes later, his mother, finally succumbing to her persistent maternal concern, tried to open the door and found her child wedged against it, collapsed and whimpering piteously. According to Carla, he had incurred a large hematoma in the fall. She reported grabbing the child off the floor and yelling out an attacking rebuke to the nanny in her panic. This understandable reaction likely further frightened the child and caused Carla to neglect his immediate need for gentle, quiet soothing.

At age three, Pedro had another fall after climbing onto a folding ladder that his older brother had carelessly left unattended. The ladder collapsed as he got to the third rung, throwing Pedro backward onto the ground. The impact of the accident on the child was twofold, with the back of his head hitting the floor and the heavy ladder striking him in the face.

Finally, at the age of eight, Pedro fell yet again. This time he was thrown from a car moving at approximately twenty-five miles per hour. He sustained yet another head injury, as well as deep abrasions across both shoulders. The seriousness of this fall occasioned a weeklong stay in the hospital, with three initial days of isolation in the intensive care unit. Pedro's tics appeared two months after this third fall.

As we started the session, it was obvious to me that Pedro was uncomfortable in this group setting, as he was fidgeting and glancing furtively around the room. I noticed that he was intermittently clenching his fist and drew his attention to this gesture. I asked him to see if he could begin to feel the sensations of the clenching by "putting his mind right into his fist." This wording helped Pedro learn to discern the difference between *thinking about* his hand and actually *observing it as physical sensation.* Such a shift in perspective can be quite elusive at first, but often arrives suddenly as a "mini-revelation." This new vantage brings with it an excitement, as though learning a new language and being able to communicate with the locals for the first time; here, however, the foreign language was the interoceptive (interior) landscape of the body and the local resident was the core, primal ("authentic") Self.

I observed a nascent curiosity in Pedro and asked him to *slowly* close his hand and then *slowly* open it as he put his direct (sensate) awareness into this continuous movement.* "So now, Pedro," I asked, "how does it feel when it is closed into a fist, and then how does it feel when it is slowwwly opened?"

"Hmm," he responded. "My fist feels strong, like I can stand up for myself."

---

* The emphasis of this slow, deliberate, mindful inner movement contrasts with what is frequently asked for in various expressive therapies, such as "psychodrama" or some Gestalt therapies. These therapies tend to accentuate gross external movement rather than internal, *felt,* movement. These inner movements are more involuntary and employ different brain systems, including the brain stem, cerebellum, and extrapyramidal systems.

"OK," I replied, "that's great, Pedro; and now how does it feel when it's opening?"

At first, Pedro was bewildered by my question, but then he smiled. "It feels like I want to receive something for myself ... something that *I* want. It feels like I really want to get over my panic attacks so I can go to Disneyland."

"And how does that *wanting* feel to you right now?" I asked.

He paused and then replied, "It's funny—my fist feels like it has the power I need to get over my problems. And then when my hand opens it feels like I can use that strength to reach for it, to reach for what I want for myself."

I asked, "Is there anywhere else in your body where you feel something like that power or that reaching?"

"Well," he said, pausing for a moment, "I can also feel something like that in my chest ... it feels warm there and like I have more room to breathe."

"Can you show me with your hand where you feel that?" I asked. Pedro made a slow circular movement. As he continued, I noticed that the circle was gradually getting larger in an outward spiraling motion. "So Pedro," I asked, "Do you feel the warmth spreading?"

"Yes," he replied, "It feels like a warm sun."

"And what color is it?"

"It's yellow, like the sun ... Oh wow! Now, when I feel my hand opening, the warmth is spreading into my fingertips and they are starting to tingle."

"OK, Pedro, that's great! I think that you are now ready to face the problem."

"Yeah," he replied, "Yeah, I know it."

"And how do you know it?" I asked, tipping my head quizzically.

He giggled. "Oh, that's easy—I feel it in my body."

"OK then!" I responded encouragingly. "So then, let's go on."

We see in Figure 5.1 (see insert after page 58) that it is our present (here-and-now) somatic state that determines the relationship and platform to renegotiate a traumatic procedural memory. This initial awareness work that I had just completed with Pedro now became the embodied foundation for further investigation. The outcome of the entire session was first germinated in this initial here-and-now inner exploration. Bringing attention to Pedro's fist may seem trivial; however, it was the sensing of this *subtle inner movement,* the burgeoning awareness of how this movement really felt from the inside that set the stage for the remainder of the session. This somatically based, resourced platform made it safe enough for Pedro to now process his challenging procedural memories and then ultimately to support their transformation. It cannot be overstated how the body's felt sense allows physiological access to procedural memories. These are the crucial implicit memories that cognitive approaches simply don't engage and cathartic approaches frequently override and overwhelm.

A fundamental concept in Somatic Experiencing (SE) is *pendulation,* used in resolving implicit traumatic memories. Pendulation, a term I have coined, refers to the *continuous, primary, organismic rhythm of contraction and expansion.* Traumatized individuals are stuck in chronic contraction; in this state of fixity, it seems to them like nothing will ever change. This no-exit fixation entraps the traumatized individual with feelings of extreme helplessness, hopelessness, and despair. Indeed, the sensations of contraction seem so horrible and so endless, with no apparent relief in sight, that individuals will do almost anything to avoid feeling their bodies. The body has become the enemy. These sensations are perceived as the feared harbinger of the entire trauma reasserting itself. However, it is just this avoidance that keeps people frozen, "stuck" in their trauma. With gentle guidance, they can discover that when these sensations are "touched into," just for a few moments, they can survive the experience—they learn that they won't be annihilated. While exiting numbness and shutdown often feels more acutely disturbing at first, with gentle yet firm support people can suspend their resistance and open to a tentative curiosity. Then as these sensations are contacted, momentarily and very gradually, the contraction opens to expansion and then moves naturally back to contraction. This time, however, the contraction feels less stuck, less ominous, and then leads to another spontaneous experience of quiet expansion. With each cycle—contraction, expansion, contraction, expansion— the person begins to experience an inner sensation of *flow* and a growing sense of allowance for relaxation. With this sense of inner movement, freedom, and flow, they gradually ease out of trauma's terrifying and gripping "dragnet."

Another foundation stone in this early therapeutic exploration involves contacting both inner strength and the allied capacity for what I call *healthy aggression.** For Pedro, this initial contact occurred when he became aware of the felt strength in his fists and then the openness in his hands. Together they comprised the new experience of healthy aggression: the capacity to stand up for himself, to mobilize and direct his power toward getting what he needs, and thereby opening to new possibilities. So with this reliable, steadfast foundation, Pedro was now equipped to confront the dragons that were "dragging-on" his aliveness and forward movement in life. So what happened next?

I engaged Pedro in a series of slow, repeated *titrated,* movement exercises that involved gradually opening his mouth to the point of resistance and then gently closing it.[18] These exercises replicated his earlier exploration of contraction and expansion,

---

* The word "aggression" derives from the Latin verb *aggredi*, which can mean "to approach," "to have a goal," "to seize an opportunity," or "to desire," among other things.

and interrupted Pedro's compulsive "over-coupled" sequence of neuromuscular contractions in his head, neck, and jaw. A rest between each set of these openings and closings allowed for an interlude of settling, a periodic quieting of his arousal. As Pedro moved through these graduated efforts, he experienced some abrupt shudders in his neck and shoulder, and then a softer trembling (a "discharging") in his legs during the resting phase.[19] He also reported an uncomfortable and intense burning heat that emanated from the tops of his shoulders. This "body memory," his mother later observed, was located where the lacerations from his third childhood fall had left considerable scarring. After several more cycles of micro-movement/discharge/rest, Pedro's tics were significantly reduced and he was clearly more present and available for interaction with me, as his "guide," and the class as his supportive allies.

As the tic movements subsided, Pedro reported feeling much more at ease. I then asked him what *he* wanted most from the session. He offered that he was really hoping to get rid of his claustrophobic fears so that he could travel with his family from Brazil to Disneyland for spring vacation. He told me that previously he had experienced a panic attack when he was in a hot, stuffy plane that got delayed at the gate, held in waiting for over thirty minutes with its doors sealed shut. I asked him what he noticed when he thought about being in the plane.

"Scared," he murmured.

"And how does that feel in your body?"

"Like I can't really breathe ... like there's a band around my chest ... I really can't breathe." I put my foot next to Pedro's, asking first if that would be OK. "Yes," he responded, "it helps me not go away into the air."

With this added "grounding," I asked Pedro whether the tension in his chest had become stronger or weaker, stayed the same, or if it had changed to something else. This type of *open questioning* evoked a stance of curiosity on Pedro's part. He paused for a few moments and then offered, "It's definitely getting better. It feels like I can take a breath."

"Is there anything else that you notice?" I asked.

"Yes," he replied "I feel some warmth in my chest again … and it's starting to spread up into my face.*

"Yeah," he added "it's really spreading now, moving through the rest of my body … it feels really good, like warm tingles and a gentle shaking … and inner shaking … that's really funny … it's like the panic went away, like it's gone … like it's really gone!"

I asked Pedro if he could recall another recent experience involving his claustrophobic panic. He described an occasion a year earlier when he was playing in a swimming pool with a large ball that could be entered into through a zippered opening. Once a person was inside, the ball could be closed from within by pulling up on the zipper. The passenger could then roll the ball across the surface of the water by shifting his weight. This ball was meant to create fun and excitement. Pedro, however, was not having fun. Instead, the closed interior was stifling to him and he fell backward. This re-created the terrifying interoceptive experience of his previous falls, as well as the suffocation panic he had experienced when he was caught in the airplane. Pedro panicked when he could not open the ball. Though unable to scream because of his hyperventilated breathing, his stifled moans did, once again, alert his mother. While unzipping the ball from the outside and freeing her son from his predicament, she felt an anguish similar to that which had been provoked by the strangulated moans of her injured seven-month-old baby. When Pedro emerged from this ensnaring cocoon, he saw,

---

* This corresponded visibly to a mild vasodilation in his throat and face, as observed by the "glowing" color tone of his skin.

Present Fearful State encoded, Interoceptively, as Somatic Markers*

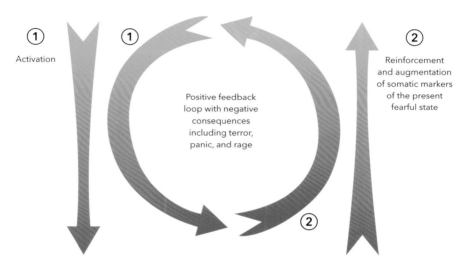

Memory Engrams with Similar Somatic Markers

* Includes: muscle tension; constriction; vibration; shaking; weakness; increased (or decreased) heart rate; increased blood pressure (pounding); low blood pressure (dizziness); fainting or light headedness; cold, sweaty hands; hypo (shallow) or hyper (over) respiration.

Figure 5.1 Somatic Markers. The above graphic illustrates how our present interoceptive state links to emotional and procedural memories exhibiting similar states. Our current physical/physiological and emotional response unconsciously guides the type of memories and associations that will be recalled; present states of fear evoke fear-based memories, which in turn reinforce the present agitated state. This can lead to a positive ("runaway") feedback loop of increasing distress and potential retraumatization.

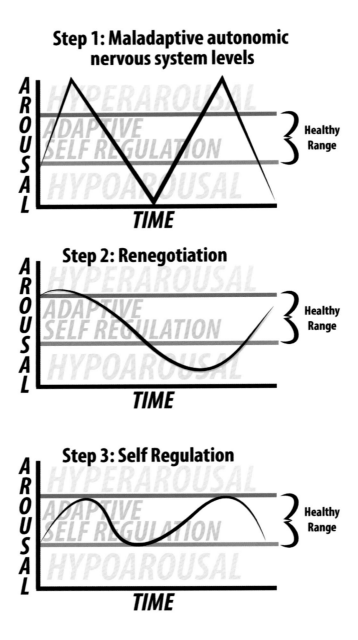

Figure 5.2 Window of Self-Regulation. The above charts show the renegotiation of hyperarousal (overwhelm) states and hypoarousal (shutdown) states in re-establishing the range of self-regulation and restoring dynamic equilibrium.

again, his mother's frightened face. Her terrified expression startled him once again, intensifying his feeling of fear and defeat.

As Pedro completed his rendering of this most recent panic episode, I noted that he was slumped over in his chair. It was as though his shoulders had hunched forward and his middle spine had collapsed over his diaphragm. This sunken posture mirrored the abject shame, despair, and overwhelming passivity of his rescue—both as an adolescent and as an infant. Recognizing a timely opportunity to help Pedro experience some agency in his body, I brought his attention to his fist, which he was once again subconsciously opening and closing. "Hmm," he replied, "I can feel some of the strength here; it's coming back. It reminds me of when we first started the session." I then guided him to sense his posture and to gently deepen his forward slump. This sinking collapse came to rest, and then a spontaneous gradual upward rebound movement began. I encouraged him to simply notice his felt experience as his spine lengthened and his head lifted upward. This conscious encounter conveyed an unexpected sense of pride, or even triumph, which he acknowledged with these words: "Wow, that feels a lot better, like I can hold my head up and look ahead; it makes me feel more confident."

Building on this burgeoning exhilaration, I asked Pedro if he would be willing to revisit his most recent moment of defeat. He agreed. I suggested that he picture himself inside the ball. He seemed ready to engage in this challenging somatic visualization. He described entering the ball, closing the zipper, and then losing his balance as he started to fall backward. As he recalled this series of events, his embodied imagination led to a reexperiencing of the vertigo. This dizziness had previously ignited the initial phase of a panic reaction, including a tightening of his chest and hyperventilation. This, in turn, amplified his panicky feelings of suffocation. However, he was now able to experience it *without feeling overwhelmed.* I guided him to once again attend to the specific sensations of constriction around his chest, and his breathing gradually settled and he took several spontaneous, slow, and easy breaths with full exhalations.

We then explored his sensation of falling backward. I gently supported Pedro's upper back and head with my hands, while encouraging him to surrender and let go into the sensations of falling. He immediately reported that he "needed to get out!"

I responded calmly with the question, "And how can you do that?"

To this he replied, "It feels like I am leaving my body."

"OK," I answered, "let's just see where you go."

He acknowledged that he was afraid to give into "this weird floating feeling." Pausing to provide reassurance, I gently encouraged him to notice the floating sensations and asked him where he might float to. When this kind of dissociation occurs, it is important not to ask body-based language questions, but rather to accept and follow the dissociated experience. Pedro hesitated and then said, "Up—up out of the ball."

"Well, that might be a good place to be," I suggested.

He then described looking down at the ball from above and also knowing that he was inside of it.

I inquired, "OK, what might you want to do from up there?"

He replied, "I would like to go down and open the zipper." Even though Pedro was partially dissociated, he was able to envision and execute, in his imagination, this *active (motoric) escape* strategy. Previously, he had to rely on his mother to rescue him— hardly an empowering experience, particularly for an adolescent. This "renegotiation" led to a further reduction of his tics.

Pedro then recalled an earlier time when he'd had a similar experience. He told me that when he was five years old, the door to his bedroom got stuck and would not open. He remembered pulling at it with all of his might, to no avail. He recalled that this had precipitated a terrifying panicky reaction, like what had happened in the airplane. As therapeutic observers, we can see how this was a "replay," an echo, of his earliest experience of being hurt, helpless, and alone at seven months old. Falling out of his crib, being unable to get to his mother, and then being alone for twenty minutes (an eternity for a baby) had branded him with this searing and enduring emotional and procedural imprint.

As such, Pedro's five-year-old panicky "overreaction" to the stuck bedroom door is more than likely due to that earlier (seven-month-old) fall with its serious injury, extreme helplessness, and thwarted efforts to solicit timely attention. However, with the one success in embodied imagery of getting out of the ball under his belt, and with a relaxed determination in his jaw from the jaw awareness exercise, I had the sense that he would be able to complete his five-year-old escape from the bedroom in a way that he had not been able to accomplish previously. I felt that he would persevere and not be defeated this time.

I now asked Pedro to continue imagining pulling at the door knob and urged him to feel his whole body as he engaged in this assertive effort. When I inquired about a brief flicker of a smile that flitted across his face, he boldly described how he pulled and pulled and kicked and finally broke the door down. He then smiled broadly and I asked him where he could feel that Cheshire grin. "Oh," he replied, "I can really feel it in my eyes, my arms, my chest, shoulders, legs, and even here," he said, pointing to his belly. "Really all over my body. I feel super strong and powerful, like a superhero ... my body can protect me," he offered triumphantly.

Like many parents, Pedro's mother had reported that she was concerned about her teenage boy's excessive use of the computer and internet; it did appear that his usage was extreme and compulsive. Two days after our session, she reported that Pedro had asked her to buy him some art supplies. He used to enjoy drawing as a child, but after his symptoms had worsened and involved his face, head, and neck, he had lost all interest in art and became glued to the computer. This compulsion seemed to make his symptoms worse. She was more than a little pleased with this new artistic development. And then to her complete surprise he took the bold initiative of joining a singing class at his school. There he could feel the powerful connection between his jaw and diaphragm. Pedro also relayed to his mother that he had a new plan for his future schooling, stating that he wanted to do research in the field of psychology instead of his earlier choice of engineering. He was fascinated by what was going on in his own brain and was eager to do the brain scan that they had put off for years because his claustrophobia was so severe. Pedro now expressed excitement about planning the family trip to Disneyland. Apprehension about the long plane trip seemed to have disappeared. This most certainly was a new multidimensional change of perspective on his future—a future very different from his past. So let us now briefly summarize the steps of renegotiation that brought Pedro to his new, updated memories and how they enabled Pedro to put his past behind him and then move forward, empowered and self-directed.

To summarize, the basic steps in renegotiating a traumatic memory generally involve these processes:

1. Help create a here-and-now experience of relative calm presence, power, and grounding. In this state the client is taught how to visit his positive body sensations, as well as his difficult, traumatically based sensations.

2. Using this calm, embodied platform, the client is directed to gradually shift back and forth between the positive, grounded sensations and the more difficult ones.

3. Through this sensate tracking, the traumatic procedural memory emerges in its traumatic, truncated (i.e., thwarted) form. The therapist continues to check that the client is not in an over-activated (or under-activated) state. If they are, the therapist returns to the first two steps.

4. Having accessed the truncated form of the procedural memory, the therapist, recognizing the "snapshot" of the failed (i.e., incomplete) response, encourages further sensate exploration and development of this protective action through to its intended and meaningful completion.

5. This leads to a resetting of the core regulatory system, restoring balance, equilibrium, and relaxed alertness.[20] (See Figure 7.1, page 132.)

6. Finally, the procedural memories are linked with the emotional, episodic, and narrative functions of memory. This allows the memory to take its rightful place where it belongs—in the past. The traumatic procedural memories are no longer being reactivated in their maladaptive (incomplete) form, but are now transformed as empowered healthy agency and triumph. The entire structure of the procedural memory has been changed, promoting the emergence of new (updated) emotional and episodic memories.

A key feature in working with traumatic memories is to visit them incrementally from the vantage of a present state which is neither a state of hyper-activation and overwhelm nor a state of shutdown, collapse, and shame. This can be a bit confusing for therapists, because individuals who are in a state of shutdown may *appear* to be calm.

In general when working with procedural memories, it is best to work with the more recent ones first. In reality, however, all procedural memories with similar elements and attendant states of consciousness tend to merge into a composite procedural engram. Pedro's explicit recall of being trapped in the ball allowed him to access the procedural engram of being helplessly trapped and then to engineer an active escape. The full renegotiation of the composite engram was accomplished, so to speak, retrospectively. This allowed Pedro to find completion, first in freeing himself from the ball as an adolescent and then in opening the door as a five-year-old. These two discreet phases of his session also helped address the composite engram that included his pervasive feelings of helplessness as an infant. Hence, his primal infantile anguish was also neutralized to some degree along with the successful reworking of his adolescent and five-year-old traumas.

Pedro's form of triumph was also manifested in a session I had with a champion marathon runner who was dealing with intimacy problems related to her childhood sexual abuse by an uncle. In her session, she experienced the impulse to fight back and kick him in the genitals. She also recognized (with a growing self-compassion) that he had, in fact, fully overpowered her as a four-year-old. After that, she then felt her power returning, as she imagined extending her arms as a form of boundary against his advances. At the end of the session, she reported feeling like she had run a marathon. I asked her what that felt like, to which she replied: "It felt like I was getting to a point where my legs were going to give out; they felt like I could barely stand, no less continue to run … and then something happened. It was like I heard a voice in my head saying, 'Just keep moving … keep moving.'"

I asked her if that was a common experience for long-distance runners. "Yes," she replied, "but in our session, I was feeling that from the inside, inside the whole of me, not just in my legs. I can defend myself now; I know I have this capacity for enduring great challenges and overcoming obstacles."

She told me a week later that she had experienced some opening to sexual intimacy—and this, she added, "was her greatest triumph over him [her uncle]."

On the Will to Persevere

The world breaks everyone and
afterward many are strong in the broken places.
—ERNEST HEMINGWAY

You gain strength, courage, and confidence
by every experience in which you really stop to look fear in the face.
You are able to say to yourself, "I have lived through this horror.
I can take the next thing that comes along."
You must do the thing you think you cannot do.
—ELEANOR ROOSEVELT, *YOU LEARN BY LIVING: ELEVEN KEYS FOR A*
MORE FULFILLING LIFE

My forty-five years of clinical work confirms a fundamental and universal instinct geared toward overcoming obstacles and restoring one's inner balance and equilibrium: an instinct to persevere and to heal in the aftermath of overwhelming events and loss. In addition, I suspect that this instinct has physical footprints in a biological rooted will to persevere and triumph in the face of challenge and adversity. Any therapist worth his or her fees not only recognizes this primal capacity to meet adverse challenges, but also understands that their primary role is not to "counsel," "cure," or "fix" their clients, but rather to support this innate drive for perseverance and triumph. But how do we facilitate the fulfillment of this instinct?

I will freely admit that this inner quest for transformation, illustrated by Pedro's journey, portrays a drive, the nature of which I have reflected upon and pondered for many of these years. Recently a German colleague, Joachim Bauer, knowing of my investigations, handed me an obscure journal article based on the treatment of a few epileptic patients. However, before we discuss this interesting paper, let me first offer a short background on the neurosurgical treatment of epilepsy.

Since the pioneering work of the eminent mid-twentieth-century neurologist Wilder Penfield, a procedure for remediating severe, intractable epilepsy involved cutting out the brain cells that are damaged, thus averting these violent "nerve storms." However, before this surgical extirpation proceeds, the neurosurgeon must first establish what the afflicted brain region controls or processes. This is done so that the surgeons do not inadvertently cut out and interfere with a function vital to that individual. Since there are no pain receptors in the brain, this procedure is readily done with the patient fully awake and responsive as the surgeon stimulates these focal areas with an electrode probe.

Until recently, most of these electrical stimulations have been confined to the surface of the brain and have been associated with specific concrete functions. For example, if somato-sensory areas are stimulated, patients generally report sensations in various parts of their body. Or if the motor cortex is stimulated, then a part of the body, such as a finger, moves in response to the electrical stimulus. Penfield also reported that there were some "associational" areas (including the hippocampus) that, when he stimulated them, the person reported dreamlike reminiscences. Some sixty-five years later, after these initial investigations, protocols were developed to position electrodes in various deep brain areas for the same purpose of treating intractable epilepsy.

In the provocative case study handed to me by my German friend, a group of Stanford researchers published an article with the intriguing title "The Will to Persevere Induced by Electrical Stimulation of the Human Cingulate Gyrus."[21] It reported on an unexpected experience provoked by the delivery of deep brain stimulation to a completely different part of the brain than had been previously explored by Penfield and other earlier neurosurgeons.

This brain region is known as the *anterior midcingulate cortex* (aMCC).

The patients in this study experienced something quite remarkable. The exact words of patient number two, as his aMCC was stimulated, were: "I'd say it's a question ... not a worry like a negative ... it was more of a positive thing like ... to push harder, push harder, push harder to try and get through this ... if I don't fight, I give up. I can't give up ... I (will) go on." Patient one described his experience with this metaphor: "It's like you were driving a car into a storm and ... like one of the tires was half-flat ... and you're only halfway there and you have no other way to go back ... you just have to keep going forward." Both patients in the study recounted a sense of "challenge" or "worry" (known as foreboding), *yet remained motivated and prepared for action, aware that they would overcome the challenge.* Wow!

During the stimulation of these patients, the authors noted increases in heart rate, while at the same time the patients reported autonomic signs including "shakiness" and "hot flashes" in the upper chest and neck region. Indeed, for me this rang a thunderous bell, as most of my clients have reported very similar autonomic sensations as they worked with their traumatic procedural memories and moved from fear through arousal and mobilization into triumph. At the same time, my clients exhibited subtle postural changes including an extension of the spine and an expansion of the chest.

From a physiological point of view, there is at the level of the aMCC a functional convergence of the (dopamine-mediated) systems for *motivation* and the (noradrenergic) one for *action*. To keep things in perspective, let us not forget that for thousands of years, well before the advent of neuroscience, such triumphant convergence of motivation and action, of focus and the will to persevere, has been described in numerous myths from around the world and in our everyday lives. From a mythological vantage, these researchers and their courageous patients may have just uncovered a neurological substrate of the "hero's journey."

In his landmark book *The Hero with a Thousand Faces*, the eminent mythologist Joseph Campbell traces the occurrence of this myth throughout the world and across recorded history. He makes a compelling case that it is precisely this coming to terms with one's destiny, through meeting a great challenge (whether external or internal) and then mastering it with clear direction, courage, and perseverance, that is at the core of this universal archetype, the hero/heroine myth. This perseverance in meeting extreme adversity is also the basis of many shamanic initiation rituals. The will to persevere, this initiation or trial by fire, may be exactly what this sliver of brain tissue—the aMMC—seems to orchestrate. Indeed, it may be part of the core neural architecture facilitating triumph over adversity, the quintessential encounter of the human condition. Clinically, we need to address the central question of how that part of the brain normally gets stimulated in the absence of epilepsy and depth electrodes.

Current research on the aMCC shows that this brain region is activated when there are stimuli of strong affective salience, whether positive or negative. It has clear neural connections with areas in the insula, amygdala, hypothalamus, brain stem, and thalamus. The aMCC, along with the insula cortex, receives its primary input from sense receptors inside the body. In addition, it is the only part of the cortex that can actually dampen the amygdala's fear response.[22] Indeed, this circuit of thalamus, insula, anterior cingulate, and the medial prefrontal Cortex receives interoceptive information, i.e., involuntary internal body sensations, and affects the preparation for action via the extrapyramidal motor system. These are the very fabric of which procedural memories are made.[23] (See Figure 7.1, page 132.)

Without the benefit of a multimillion-dollar brain scanner, we are free to speculate on the two-way communication between Pedro's brain and body as his internal body sensations change from ones of fear and helplessness to those of triumph and mastery. To this end I wish to enlist the existence of a crucial "instinct": an innate somatic drive to overcome adversity and move forward in life. Indeed, without this primal instinct, trauma therapy would be limited to insight and cognitive behavioral interventions, whereas with this instinct engaged, transformation becomes possible as the client gradually meets and embraces trauma. I further speculate that this instinct operates through activating the coordinated, procedurally based systems for motivation, reward, and action. This convergence of motivation and action systems (dopamine and nor-adrenaline) is what I have called "healthy aggression."

A few case studies on the deep brain stimulation of epileptic patients can hardly be considered proof of the existence of an instinct to persevere and triumph. However, a body of clinical evidence (as I describe in *In An Unspoken Voice),* as well as the accumulation of world myths, rituals, and a multitude of films and written literature, speaks to the universality of perseverance and triumph over obstacles and challenges as being at the heart of human endeavors. Perhaps this hard-wiring for transformation not only speaks to our humanity but also connects us to our ancestors, both human and animal.

Indeed, in the session with Pedro, we saw how the *access and completion of his procedural memories* was the therapeutic pathway toward confronting and transmuting his demons and then to "mythically" fulfilling his rite of passage as he transformed these procedural memories from helpless child to competent adult. Thus, he begins to assume the mantle of his destiny as a potent and autonomous young man.

Insula, aMCC, and Ecstasy—A Spiritual Side of Transforming Trauma

Fyodor Dostoevsky, who suffered from grand mal seizures, wrote of his experience in words which might seem fanciful: "A happiness unthinkable in the normal state and unimaginable for anyone who hasn't experienced it ... I am then in perfect harmony with myself and the entire universe." These sensations seemed to inform his epic novel *The Idiot,* whose central character, Prince Myshkin, says of his attacks, "I would give my whole life for this one instant."

The question about how wide ranging these "peak" experiences are among other "sufferers" has been difficult to ascertain, perhaps because people fear that they would be considered "crazy." However, a few neurologists have found what is referred to as "the Dostoevsky effect" to be a fascinating, if not legitimate, area of study. In epilepsy treatments similar to the Stanford group's stimulation of the aMCC, neurologists at the University Hospital of Geneva in Switzerland seem to have localized the initial focus of a subpopulation of their patients with "ecstatic seizures."[24] Using powerful brain imaging techniques for detecting location of activity, they reported that the insula seems to be the focal region. In stimulating the anterior insula, they were able to evoke "spiritual rapture" in a few of their patients. It is noteworthy that when one of the patients was told she could probably be cured of her epilepsy, were she willing to forfeit these ecstatic states, she boldly and summarily declined. Even with her severe epilepsy, "it was not worth the trade-off."

The insula is divided into posterior (back) and anterior (front) sections. It appears that the posterior part registers raw ("objective") sensations, both internally and externally generated. In contrast, the anterior portion (which is associated with the aMCC) seems to process more refined, nuanced, and subjective feeling-based sensations and emotions. Craig,[25] Critchley,[26] and others have suggested that the anterior insula is largely responsible for how we feel *about* our body and ourselves. Furthermore, they note, the left side of the insula is related to positive feelings and the right side to negative ones. Once again, it is the part of the brain that receives input from interoceptive (internal body) sensors. In this regard, various spiritual traditions have developed breathing, movement, and meditative techniques to evoke these types of spiritual states while also providing guidance on how to deal with the polarity of these emotional and sensation-based states—that when one experiences ecstasy, there is a subsequent "let down," a swing to the negative realms.

In renegotiating trauma via Somatic Experiencing, we utilize "pendulation," the shifting of body sensations or emotions between those of expansion and those of contraction. This ebb and flow allows the polarities to gradually be integrated. It is the holding together of these polarities that facilitates deep integration and often an "alchemical" transformation.

What follows in Chapter 6 is a textual and visual demonstration of the role of procedural memories in trauma resolution, taken from videos of sessions with two clients. The first sequence shows a fourteen-month-old toddler named Jack. Because of his age and verbal development, his work involves only procedural and emotional memories. However, when he returns two-and-a-half years later for a follow-up, we see how the procedural memory has evolved into an episodic one.

The second session involves work with a Marine named Ray who was hit by blasts from two IEDs in Afghanistan after having his best friend die in his arms. After he resolves the procedural memories of the blast (shock trauma), he is then able to access and process his emotional, episodic, and narrative (declarative) memories, and comes to a deeper peace with his survivor's guilt, grief, and his loss of community.

TWO CASE STUDIES:
AN INTIMATE VISIT

Baby Jack

A mother and child reunion.

Jack is a bright and energetic toddler, yet at the same time painfully shy and reserved. He had been referred to me by a colleague because he had struggled through a very difficult birth and was now contending with the sequelae to that ordeal. Jack had been in a breach position with the umbilical cord wrapped three times around his neck and his head caught high in the apex of the uterus. Each push he directed with his tiny feet and legs drove his head into a tighter wedge, while further constricting the cinch around his throat; this was a "no exit" ordeal evoking a primal suffocation terror, something difficult for most adults to comprehend.[27] During the emergency C-section, doctors noted Jack's serious distress; his heart rate had dropped precipitously, indicating a life-threatening situation. In addition to the C-section, it required forceful suctioning to dislodge Jack's head from the uterine apex. His arrival into this world was accompanied by multiple clinicians poking and prodding at him, plying their trade with the necessary needle sticks, IV insertions, aggressive examinations, and rushed interventions.

Now fourteen months old, Jack was being worked up for yet another invasive procedure to investigate a condition of intermittent gastric reflux. His mother, Susan, was dutifully following through with the pediatrician's recommendations and had scheduled an endoscopy for two weeks from the day of our first session. While she appreciated the pediatrician's thoroughness, Susan was hoping that there might be another solution, one that was not invasive and potentially traumatizing. With this hope in tow, she and her young son arrived on my doorstep late in the fall of 2009.

Jack sat astride his mother's hip as I opened the door and interrupted her second knock. She looked somewhat abashed as the follow-through on her rapping propelled her across the threshold and into my office. Regaining her composure and adjusting her son's position, she introduced herself and Jack. As they came through the entryway, I noticed an awkwardness in the shared balance of mother and son. I could have dismissed this as a general unease with a new environment, an unfamiliar stranger, and an unknown form of therapy. However, it seemed to be more fundamental than that; there was a basic discordance in their dyadic rhythm.

It is often assumed that when there is a disconnection between baby and mother, there was a failure on the part of the caregiver to provide the "good enough" environment required for bonding. This is not always true, as, clearly, was the case with Susan. She earnestly and lovingly provided comfort, support, and attention. It was, rather, the traumatic birth that caused a jolt, splitting them apart at birth. The subsequent "shock wave" disturbed their mutual capacity to participate in each other's most intimate moments, to fully bond and attach.

In my office, Jack scanned his new surroundings as his mother summarized his symptoms and the upcoming procedure. While concurring with her concern and offering information about how I work, I was also tuning into her son's here-and-now process. Following his gaze, I could see that he was intrigued with the colorful array of toys, musical instruments, dolls, and sculptures that were crowded onto the shelves above my table.

I picked out a turquoise Hopi gourd rattle and began slowly shaking its seeds. Using the rhythm to engage baby and mom, I made eye contact with Jack and called out his name. "Hi, Jack," I intoned in rhythm with the rattle.

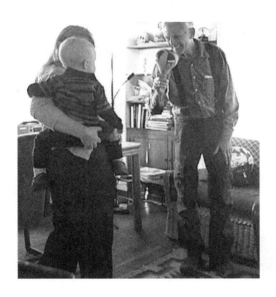

Jack tentatively reached out for it, and I slowly extended my arm to offer the handle to him. He then pulled back in response to my overture.

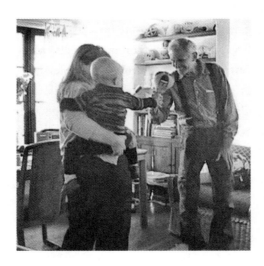

He then reached for it again with an open palm, but on contact, he pushed it away and turned toward his mother with a faint cry of distress.

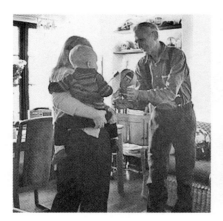
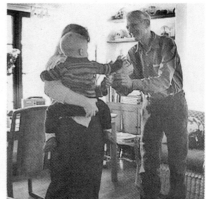

She responded by securing her hold on him and rotating away from the interaction with a quick spin. He was distracted, looked away, and became quiet. I began talking to Jack about his difficult birth, speaking as if he could understand my words. My prosody and tone modulations seemed to give him some comfort and reassurance, conveying that I was an ally and somehow understood his plight.

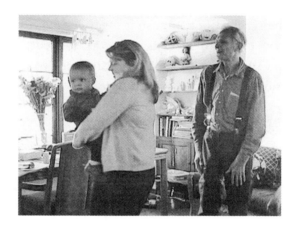

Recovering, he reached out again with curiosity and then pointed toward the table. "Apple, apple," he said, extending his left arm toward a plate holding three pomegranates.

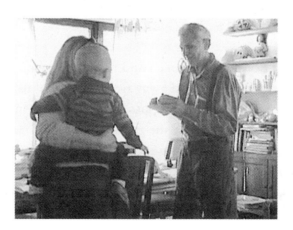

I lifted the plate and offered them to him. Jack reached for them, touched one, and then pushed it away. This time his push was more assertive. "You're into pushing, aren't you?" I asked, again communicating not only with words but with rhythm and tone. "I sure can understand how you might want to push, after all those strange people were poking and hurting you." Wanting to reinforce his pushing impulse and his power, I offered my finger to him; he reached out to push it away. "Yeah, that's great," I responded, conveying my feelings of encouragement, warmth, and support. "You sure want to get that away from you, don't you?" Jack let go another whimper, as if he agreed.

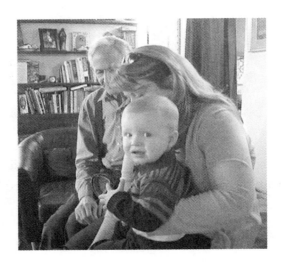

Susan sat down on the couch and began removing Jack's shoes. He seemed fearful and turned away from the two of us as we talked about his gastric reflux and its possible penetration into his lungs. When Susan mentioned that the pediatric surgeon was proposing an endoscopy, Jack seemed to show a flash of distress: His face scrunched downward in a frown of worry and anxiety as he called out, "Mama." Jack seemed to have recognized the meaning of our words (or was perhaps picking up on his mother's unease), and in a millisecond, his mid-back stiffened.

He turned toward his mother and I gently placed my hand on his mid-back, resting my palm over his stiffened and contracted muscles while extending my fingers upward between his shoulder blades.

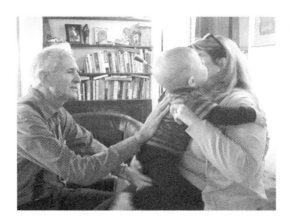

Jack whimpered again and then turned to look directly at me. Given that he maintained our eye contact, I assessed that it was safe to proceed with the physical touch. Jack continued to connect with me visually as his mother recounted the history of his symptoms, treatment, and medical assessment.

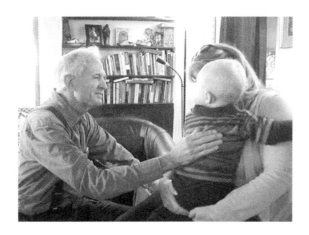

Suddenly, Jack pushed mightily against his mother's thighs with his feet and legs, propelling him upward toward her left shoulder. This movement gave me a quick snapshot of his incomplete propulsive birth movements. These were the instinctual movements (the procedural memories) that had driven him into the apex of her uterus and strangled his throat with the cord—exacerbating his distress while further activating his drive to push, creating, in turn, even more distress. As if following a dramatic, choreographed script, Jack pushed hard against his mother's legs twice more, propelling him, again, up to her shoulders.

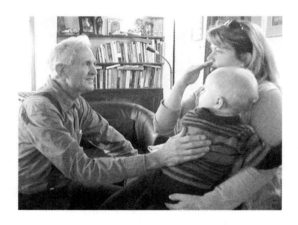

This *completion* of his birth push, without the resulting strangulation, intense cranial pressure, and "futility" brought on by his head wedging into the uterine apex, was an important sequence of movements for Jack to experience. It allowed him a successful "renegotiation"—in the here and now—of his birth process. His procedural memories shifted from maladaptive and traumatic to ones that were empowering and successful. Maintaining a low to moderate level of activation in this "renegotiation" was essential. I quietly removed my hand from his back and allowed him to settle.

His mother responded to his thrusts by standing him up in her lap. While I maintained a soft presence with an attentive, engaged gaze, Jack looked directly at me with a fierce intensity that seemed to express his furious determination. His spine elongated and he seemed both more erect and alert.*

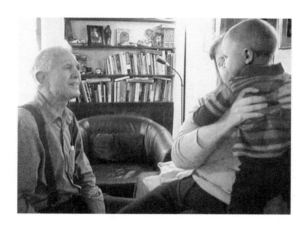

I again reached for Jack's mid-back and spoke soothingly: "I wish we had more time to play, but since they are planning this procedure in a few weeks, I want to see if we can do something to help you." Jack stiffened again and strongly pushed my hand away with his. He grimaced and flashed me a look of snarling anger while simultaneously retracting his hand and priming for another major defensive push away.

---

* In my clinical work, I have observed that children who were born via C-section often have a lack of power when they first attempt standing as toddlers. Then, as mature adults, they often have difficulties initiating actions in the world.

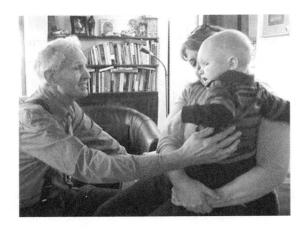

I offered Jack some resistance by bringing my thumb into the center of his small palm. By matching his force and allowing him to push me away with his strength, I observed that, as his arm extended, he was able to harness the full-throttle power of his mid-back and then follow through with a robust thrust. We maintained eye contact and I responded to his expression of concerted aggression by opening my eyes wider in surprise, encouragement, excitement, and invitation.

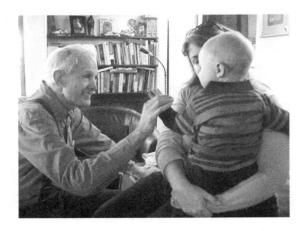

As he pushed my hand away, his response transformed into one of seeming celebration. I reflected back to him his great triumph over an unwelcomed intruder, an intruder who characterized his earliest experience of a threatening and hostile world.

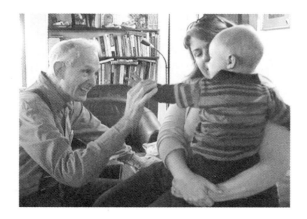

Jack pulled his hand back and let go with a small whimper, but he maintained eye contact, giving me an indication that he wanted to go on.

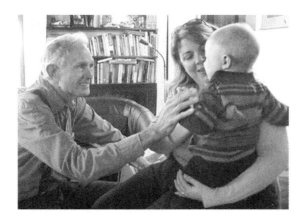

His cry strengthened as he gave one more strong push to my thumb. He howled with apparent anguish, confusion, and rage.

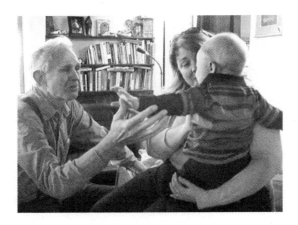

His cry deepened, becoming more spontaneous after I placed my hand on his back. This invited the sound to come through his diaphragm in deep sobs. As he pushed my hand away, once more I spoke to him about all those people touching and poking him and how much he must have wanted to push them away too.*

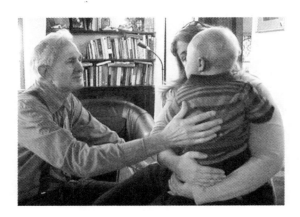

---

* While it is, of course, unlikely that Jack understood the precise meaning of my words, I believe that communicating as if he did conveyed more than the words themselves; that it was a reflection of his distress and a recognition that I "got him."

Jack broke our eye contact for the first time in this series of pushes and turned toward his mom.

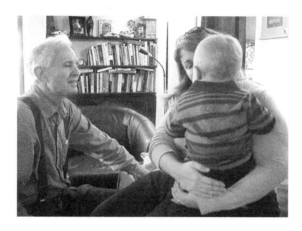

Within seconds he turned back to reengage our eye contact, even as his cry deepened. I responded to his cry with a supportive "Yeah … yeah," matching his anguish with a soothing, rhythmic prosody.

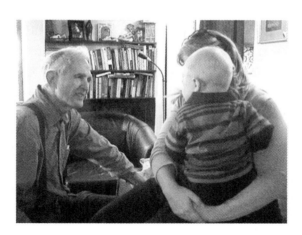

Jack took a deep and spontaneous breath for the first time, turning his chest toward his mom, then looking over his shoulder to once again return my eye contact.

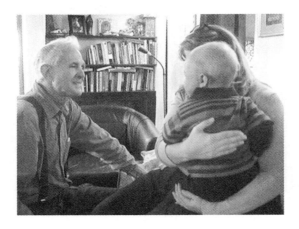

I explained to Susan about the importance of encouraging Jack's breath into the thoracic area of his back. I did this by placing my hand on hers and guiding it to his back, showing her how to support him in that area while also directing and focusing his awareness there. I explained that his pattern of tightening and constricting in this area might be in large part responsible for his reflux issues—and indeed it was! Jack continued to cry, but remained relatively relaxed. We paused for a moment, since I could see that Susan was consumed by many thoughts and feelings of her own.

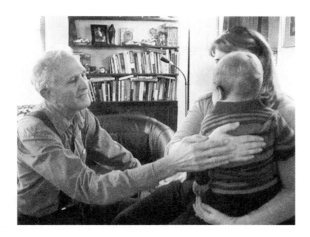

Susan took a deep breath and then looked down in amazement at her son. "He never cries," she said. "Or rather, he cries with a little whimper, but never fully like this!" I reassured her that it seemed to be a cry of deep, emotional release.

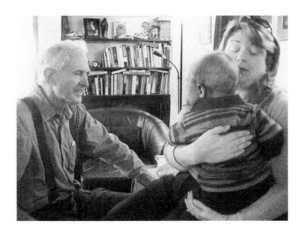

"I mean, I can't remember the last time I actually saw tears running down his face," she added in grateful astonishment.

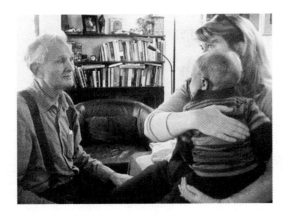

Jack reached out from his nested position and assertively pushed my finger out of the vicinity of his territory. I reinforced to Susan how profoundly disturbing it must have been for him to have strangers probing him with all those tubes and needles, how very small and helpless he must have felt. Susan repositioned herself as he burrowed deeper into her lap and chest.

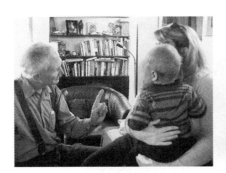 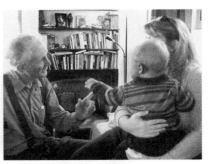

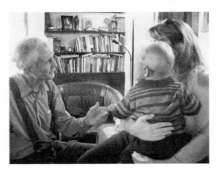

Jack nestled into his mother's lap with a new molding impulse, hitherto unseen by her. Molding is the close physical nestling of the infants' body into the shoulder, chest, and face of the mother. It is a basic component of bonding—the intimate dance that lets the infant know that he is safe, loved, and protected. I believe that it also replicates the close, contained, physical positioning of the fetus in the womb and conveys similar primal physical sensations of security and goodness.

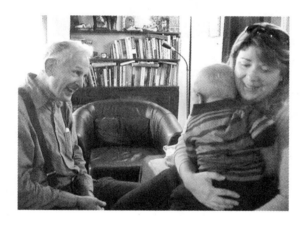

"I'm not sure what to do with this," she commented, pointing with her chin to his nuzzling and snuggling shape. We paused together for a moment to appreciate this delicate contact between the two of them.

"Whoa!" she said, breaking the silence. "He is really hot." I commented that heat was part of an autonomic discharge that accompanied his crying and emotional release.

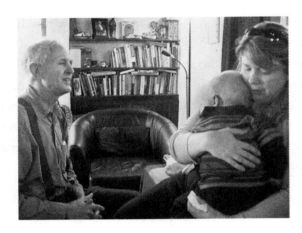

Jack settled down as she rocked him gently, maintaining full, yielding, chest-to-chest contact. He took in an easy, full inhalation and released it with a deep, spontaneous exhale that sounded both ecstatic and profoundly stress relieving. Indeed, Susan also let down her guard, shedding her doubt and beginning to trust that this new connection was "for real."

Susan looked down at her son as he continued to mold, deeply, into her chest and shoulder. She bent forward to meet his molding with her head and face. The two could be said to be "renegotiating their bonding." Susan continued to gently rock her son while maintaining their connection. He continued to regulate himself with a gentle trembling and then took several deep, spontaneous breaths with full and audible exhalations. Susan threw her head back in an ecstasy of contact and connection.

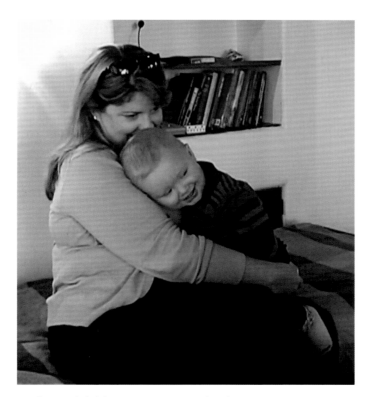

Mother and child reunion: Susan and Jack.

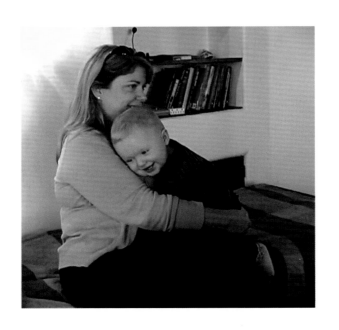

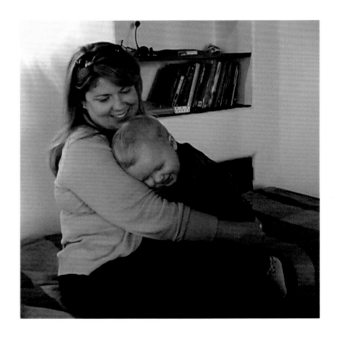

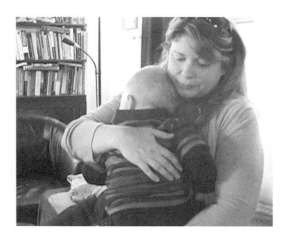

Jack peered out from his burrow and made eye contact with me. I recognized that he had had enough for one day, so I began to wind down the session. Susan acknowledged the closing, but needed to again share her own process of astonishment and hope.

With a perplexed and startled expression she noted, "I've just never seen him be this still." Then she asked Jack, "Are you asleep? So sweet, oh so sweet," as if getting to know her baby for the first time.

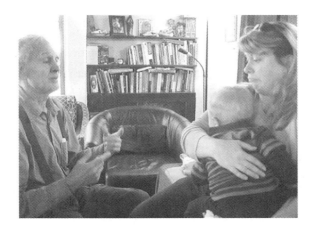

I asked Susan to take notes during the next week of anything new in Jack's behaviors, energy level, sleep patterns, reflux symptoms, and so on. Jack peeked out from his secure nesting and gave me one brief, broad smile. I responded with a return smile and a few inviting words. A couple of seconds later, another slight smile slipped across his relaxed face.

Before the end of the session, Jack and I played hide-and-seek with this warm and playful engagement for a few moments; however, at no time did he leave the cradle of his mother's lap. She nuzzled his head and mused, "This really seems different. Usually he gives a quick hug and then is off on his way." Almost as if smelling her newborn and drawing him in to her chest, she too let out an audible exhale and broke into a broad smile. "This is so very strange," she murmured quietly. "He is affectionate, but never still ... he never stays with me ... he's always off to something new."

As they continued to snuggle, they smiled in tandem. Their absolute delight was visible and palpable. Her baby had come home and they celebrated, together, that reunion.

At our next session, one week later, Susan had a number of anecdotes she wanted to share. Her upbeat excitement and Jack's comfortable curiosity were contagious. They sat down together on the couch, Jack resting his head against his mother's chest. I leaned forward in my chair, eager to hear her report. She began by recounting an episode that had occurred the night after our first session.

"He woke up in the middle of the night and called out, 'Mama,'" she reported, adding that she went to pick him up as usual. Jack sat quietly on her lap and pulled his head down deeper into her chest. "When I picked him up, he was doing this," she added, pointing with her chin to his comfortable snuggling.

I watched with an appreciative smile. "Looks to me like he's making up for lost time," I suggested.

She resumed her story: "Well … and then he said, 'Apple, apple.' I thought he wanted something to eat, but normally this would include him wiggling out of my arms and running to the kitchen. So I realized he must have been talking about the 'apples,' the pomegranates, on your table." She explained that after their last session with me, later in the week, they had an appointment with the pediatrician, which upset Jack. While they drove home in the car he kept calling out to Susan from his car seat, "Pita, pita, apple, pita."

"Again I thought he was hungry," Susan continued, "and responded by asking him if he wanted pizza. 'No,' [he answered]. 'pita, pita, apple!' I realized he was talking about you, trying to say 'Peter.' Pretty amazing, isn't it, how much he recognized and wanted to talk about the change he felt?" she queried, looking up at me for validation.*

I smiled with shared enjoyment and appreciation, and then asked about his energy. "He has been so much more talkative, much more interactive. He wants to show us lots of things and then wants our feedback. He seems much more engaged and interested in having us play with him." She bent down and kissed his head as he curled up in her lap.

"But really, this is the biggest change," she said. "I can't tell you—for him to sit and just be cuddled, it's a complete change, completely different. It's not him … it's … it's the new him."

"Or maybe it's the new us," I responded.

---

* I think Susan's report demonstrates the formation of pre-logical associational networks (procedural memory engrams), which, as we will see, remained in place when they returned for a two-year "checkup" at age four and a half.

Susan tipped her head shyly and spoke, ever so softly. "It's wonderful for me."

Jack and I played for much of the rest of this session. I recognized that much of the birth trauma and interrupted bonding was resolved and that his social engagement systems were awakening and coming online with gusto. As previously noted, the lack of attachment is far too often attributed to the mother's lack of availability and attunement. But as you can see here, it was their shared trauma that disrupted their natural rhythm and mutual drive to bond.

The molding that occurred in the first session is an essential component of bonding, a physiological "call and response" between mother and child. The renegotiation of Jack and Susan's bonding, which had been so severely interrupted by his birth crisis and neonatal care, was revisited after he discovered his capability for self-defense and the establishment of boundaries. Along with this, he had then completed the critical propulsive movements that had been overwhelmed at the time of birth and were left unresolved.

It is assumed that we have extremely limited memory of early preverbal events. However, "hidden" memory traces do exist (in the form of procedural memories) as early as the second trimester in utero and clearly around the period of birth.[28] These imprints can have a potent effect on our later reactions, behaviors, and emotional, feeling states. However, these perinatal engrams become visible only if we know where and how to look for them. A useful analogy for how to look for these deep perinatal and birth imprints, which may be obscured by later engrams, is as follows: Consider yourself sitting on the beach, observing the ocean. One becomes aware, first, of the waves and whitecaps. But then, if you were to dive in for a swim, you would be deeply affected by the currents or riptides. Indeed, they would likely have much greater impact than the waves. Further, many orders of magnitude more powerful than either of these forces are the barely visible actions of the tides. Just to recognize that they exist, we would have to sit and observe the water levels for many hours, yet the power we might capture from their force could light up an entire city.

Looking for the powerful perinatal and birth engrams beneath the more recent memory imprints requires that we clinicians use the same patient, relaxed alertness as one observing the waves, currents, and tides. As Yogi Berra said, "You can observe a lot by just watching." With Jack, these early, primal, tidal forces were noted, for example, when he propelled his whole body upward against his mother's legs as his back was supported by my hand. This action was evidence of Jack's inner drive to complete the birth movements that were thwarted when he was trapped in the apex of his mother's uterus; the more he pushed, the more trapped he became. It was the long-term outcome of his successful renegotiation of the birth traumas that we observed and consolidated at his follow-up visit a couple of years later.

Jack's Follow-Up Visit

To belatedly celebrate Jack's fourth birthday, I invited Susan to bring him in for a short visit. I was excited to see the two of them, both because of the delicate moments we had shared together and, quite frankly, from my curiosity about just how his procedural memories would express themselves.

Conventional understanding of neurological development posits that when I first saw Jack at the age of fourteen months, he was far too young to form any episodic or conscious memories. Furthermore, the existence of anything resembling an autobiographical and narrative memory would be impossible at this age. As they entered through my door, I reintroduced myself to Jack and

Susan. She asked him if he remembered me. He definitively declined with an emphatic "No!" However, Susan chuckled and said, "As we approached the door he asked me, 'Mama, is he going to put his hand on my back?'" Clearly, Jack had episodic access to the procedural (body-based) memory from our encounter when he was fourteen months old.

Recall that in his first session Jack was able to engage and develop the impulse to set boundaries and to no longer feel helpless. By then discovering that he could push and successfully propel himself through the birth canal, this time without getting stuck, he achieved a new mastery of the birth process. Along with the crying and autonomic discharge (waves of heat and spontaneous breaths), his and his mother's innate biological drives were prompted and united, leading to his deep molding and their bonding connection. In this sequence he was able to embody the totality of this experience that was encapsulated in the image of the pomegranate ("apple"). This seemed to reinforce his connection to the three of us. Later, he was able to call on this image and my name ("pita") to help regulate himself after being frightened by the doctor.

Now at my door, four-and-a-half-year-old Jack's procedural memory had morphed into an emotional one—the feeling of what had happened—and a desire for more of these feelings. The transformation of his memory engrams, from procedural to emotional to episodic, can be recognized in his expectant question, "Is he going to put his hand on my back?"

Susan went on to say that Jack had turned out to be a stellar athlete, as well as being one of the brightest children in his prekindergarten class. No surprise, as his interest in many of the objects in my room was enduring. She also noted that he rarely would curl up in her lap unless he was sad, tired, or scared—perfectly normal for a child his age.

"So Jack," I asked, "what is your favorite sport?"

"Baseball," he answered with a grin.

"And what position do you play?" I asked.

"Oh, I like to play pitcher and second base and also catcher," he replied, smiling with an evident pride in his ability to remember all these positions.

Susan said that he was always playing with his peers and had become quite autonomous, although she added, "He still likes to be hugged and nestled from time to time." As though on cue, Jack climbed up into his mother's lap and nuzzled his head and shoulders into her chest, just as he had done three years earlier. And just as she had done at that time, a broad smile appeared on his mother's lips and eyes. It was as though they had time traveled together in the shared celebration of our reunion. Susan then puzzled out loud, "This is very unusual—Jack is so social and always prefers to be active or with his friends."

So what can we make of all of this? I am quite sure that Jack did not "consciously" remember me (i.e., as a declarative memory), but then where did the question come from? What part of his memory had prompted him to ask her, "Is he going to put his hand on my back"? Indeed, was Jack using the more conscious part of his brain/mind to access the primal sensations (the procedural memories) that had remained latent until they were triggered at the threshold of my house?

Jack's four-and-a-half-year-old body began to replay his implicit experience from three years earlier, but this time he was able to put words to his bodily experience, to pose the question of whether I would put my hand on his back. And then, cued and primed, he replayed the procedural memory of securely resting in his mother's arms. Curling up on her lap with his back facing me, he invited me to put my hand on his spine and, once again, gently massage his now strong, athletic back as he melted into his mother's embracing arms.

And to top things off, he nestled in for a grand hug.

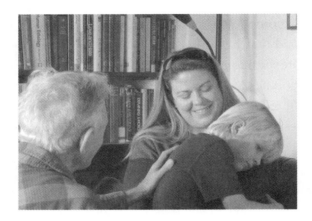

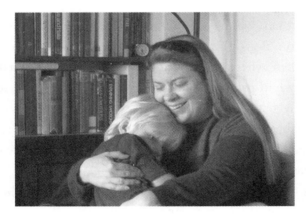

Jack continues to thrive, and I thank both him and his mother for letting me share their journey.

Ray—Healing the War Within

He who did well at war just earns the right
To begin doing well in peace.

—ROBERT BROWNING

Prologue

The cold facts: Over twenty-two suicides of military personnel occur every day. This totals more than have been killed in the entire wars in Iraq and Afghanistan, and more than twice the incidence in the general population. Ray, whose experience we shall visit, was in a platoon that had one of the highest rates of suicide in the Marine Corps.

Two to three million military personnel are returning from warfronts, bringing with them the hidden costs of war. They carry home an invisible affliction, their trauma wounds "infecting" their families and eventually their communities. Certainly if a million people returned from a warfront with an extremely virulent form of tuberculosis, it would be considered a national emergency. We would immediately summon forth the expertise and attention of scientists and clinicians throughout the country. Instead, we turn a blind eye and helplessly brace for an incoming tsunami of trauma, depression, suicide, violence, rape, divorce, addiction, and homelessness to hit our shores. The lack of effective mental health treatment for our soldiers is a broad-scale abandonment of our collective responsibilities as a nation, and particularly as therapists and healers. Neglect of these obligations almost ensures a contagious epidemic of suffering that, ultimately, affects us all.

Whatever our personal beliefs about a particular war, as a society we owe these returning warriors, who have put themselves in harm's way *in our name,* the healing and restoration to civilian life that they so deeply deserve. Ray is one of these very exceptional young veterans, and this is his story.

Ray and his platoon were stationed in Afghanistan, in the Helmand province. On June 18, 2008, they encountered a violent ambush, several of the platoon members were killed, and his best friend died in his arms. Later that day, while on patrol, two IEDs (improvised explosive devices) exploded in rapid succession. These blasts, in close proximity to Ray, literally propelled him into the air. He awoke two weeks later in the military hospital in Landstuhl, Germany, unable to walk or talk. Only gradually, and with sheer willpower, was he able to relearn those basic skills. When I first saw Ray about six months later, he was suffering greatly from symptoms of PTSD, TBI (traumatic brain injury), chronic pain, severe insomnia, depression, and what was diagnosed as Tourette's syndrome. He was on a cocktail of powerful psychiatric medications including benzodiazepines, Seroquel (an "antipsychotic"), multiple SSRIs, and opioid pain meds.

In December 2008, Ray was brought to a consultation group I was holding in Los Angeles (Session 1). After this initial session, we did three more pro-bono sessions at my home (Sessions 2, 3, and 4). And then, in 2009, I invited him to participate in a five-day workshop I was offering at the Esalen Institute in the majestic setting of the rugged Big Sur California coastline (Sessions 5 through 10). This provided an opportunity to continue our work together and gave Ray the possibility of interacting with others in a safe and supportive social environment.

Session 1

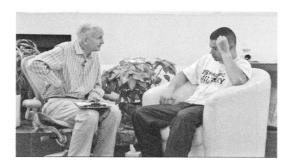

Ray began by talking about the dozen or so powerful and numbing psychiatric and narcotic medications he was taking to treat a multiplicity of diagnoses. Functionally, his impairment consisted of convulsive contractions of the head and neck, beginning first in the eyes and jaw and then spreading downward into the neck and shoulders. In this initial interview, he looked away and down at the floor, unable to make eye contact and conveying a pervasive sense of shame and defeat.

As Ray attempted to make eye contact, I noticed one of these convulsive contractions. This sequence took place in an interval of approximately one-half second and is probably the reason he was diagnosed with Tourette's. From the point of view of Somatic Experiencing, however, these rapid sequences are viewed as *incomplete orienting and defensive responses*. At the moment of the first explosion, Ray's ears, eyes, and neck would have (just barely) initiated a turn toward the source of the event. These *premotor preparatory responses* are triggered in primitive brain stem core response networks (CRNs).[29] However, well before this action was even executed, the second blast occurred almost simultaneously, and the two explosions hurled him violently into the air. At this point, his head and neck would have been pulled abruptly into his torso (the so-called turtle reflex), while the rest of his body initiated a curling up into a ball (or, to phrase it technically, he contracted in a global flexion reflex). Together, they form a snapshot of the incomplete orienting and protective defensive sequence that had become

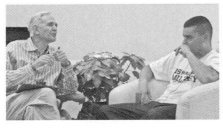

(a)

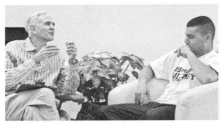

(b)

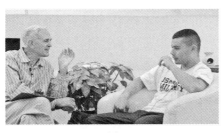

(c)

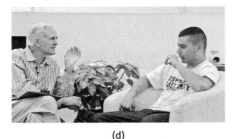

(d)

"stuck" and overwhelmed. This incomplete procedural memory (fixed action pattern) gives rise to perseveration and the so-called Tourette's-like tic spasms.

I noticed that Ray's jaw contracted first, a fraction of a second prior to the full convulsion, which involved the neck and shoulders. To interrupt this sequence, I had him very, very slowly open and close his jaw: opening to the point where he *began to feel resistance or fear* and then letting his mouth close, ever so slightly. We did this again, opening to the point where he felt the resistance, and each time gradually expanding the opening. I had him repeat this awareness exercise a few times. Each time, we saw that his mouth was able to open a small amount more. This exercise allowed the convulsive sequence to play out, at a much attenuated level by reducing this "over-coupling". Ray suddenly opened his eyes, looked around in curiosity, and described a pleasant tingling sensation spreading from his jaws into his arms.

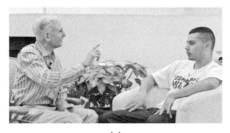

(a)

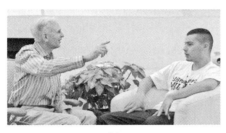

(b)

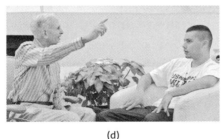

(c)

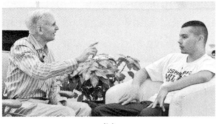

(d)

* To avoid confusion, this process of visually activating the spatial-temporal quadrant of a shock response is not related in any way to the finger movements as used in EMDR.

Next, I had Ray follow my finger with his eyes. (The elapsed time for following my finger was about 5 to 6 seconds).

Eye movements are a vital part of the orienting response. If there is a loud sound (or even the faint sound of foot-steps or the cracking of a branch in the forest), our eyes try to localize the source of the disturbance. What I was looking for in this exercise was just where his eyes, along the horizontal, vertical, or circular axes, froze, jumped, or "spaced out." Ray's eyes would have been initiating an orienting response toward the source of the first explosion, but then would have been overwhelmed, unable to lock onto and identify the source of the threat as he was blown into the air. Clearly his nervous system was unable to process this utterly overwhelming series of events which followed the fire-fight and the death of his dear friend. Uncoupling the eye movements allowed the clamping-down of his jaw muscles, which I had already identified as the initiator of his convulsive neuromuscular sequence (procedural memory) to further resolve.

In examining his visual response, I saw his eyes lock across 5 to 10 degrees in the left quadrant, reinforcing my suspicion that the blast came from his left side. I stopped my finger movement at the point where Ray's eyes froze or "spaced out." These reactions represented episodes of constriction and dissociation, respectively. When either of these outcomes occurred, I paused and allowed the activation to settle. This combination of exertion, triggered response, settling, and stabilization promotes the forward movement of the procedural memory in the direction of an eventual completion.* As I carried out this process in intervals, moving gently through activation/deactivation cycles, Ray's eye tracking began to gradually "smooth out," and the convulsive sequence softened and began to become more organized. Ray reported feeling more peaceful.

After resting for a couple of minutes, allowing his activation to settle, I continued the eye tracking. This time there was only a minute activation of the convulsive sequence. Ray then took his first easy (spontaneous) breath and his heart rate slowed from about 100 to 75. I observed this by watching the carotid artery in his neck. He described a deep relaxation in his hands and a "tingling and warmth spreading all over [his] body." The contented expression on my face reflects our shared experience of his settling as he moved toward an enjoyable tranquility.

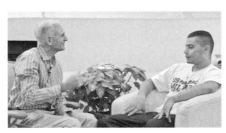

(a)

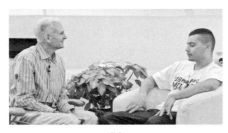

(b)

Elapsed Time ~ 10 seconds

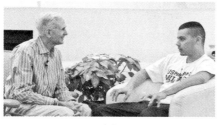

(a)

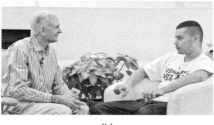

(b)

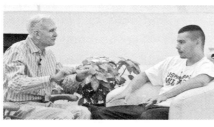

(c)

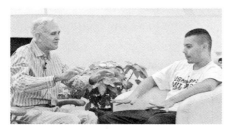

(d)

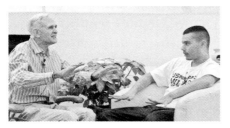

(e)

Next, Ray spontaneously stretched out his hands. I had him place his mind in his hands and to really sense what that feels like (interoceptively) from the inside. As Ray did this, each time, he gradually opened his hands wider and wider. This helped him to make greater contact with the dynamic healing rhythms of "pendulation," pulsation, and flow.

Elapsed Time
~ 5 seconds

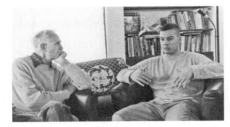

(a)

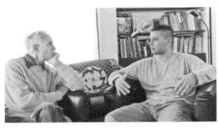

(b)

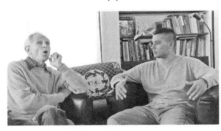

(c)

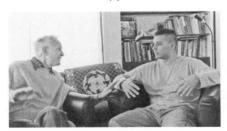

(d)

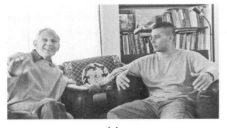

(e)

Session 3

In the third session, at my home, I asked Ray to evaluate his progress by noting where he was at this point in time on a scale of one to ten—one being where he started out before our first session in Los Angeles and ten being where he is fully competent, confident, and has the life that he wants. He reported that he was a four. I then asked if he could look ahead into the future and see where he thought that he would be in the next weeks and months. He opened his arms in an expansive gesture and then said he could see himself as a six … and then as an eight. As his "coach/guide" I didn't hide my enthusiasm at his belief in his own healing momentum. This "quantitative" assessment that Ray had so energetically participated in is a useful exercise, in that it helps to demonstrate to the client that they are clearly moving out of the traumatic shock/shutdown where they could not imagine having a future different from their (traumatic) past. As Ray so aptly put it, "Now I can see myself having a bright future."

Session 5

The next sessions with Ray took place during a one-week workshop at the Esalen Institute in Big Sur California.

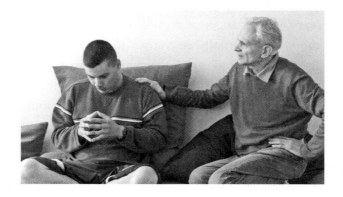

During this session I had Ray make a particular sustained "voo" sound, along with opening and closing jaw movements.* This was to help connect his vital energy center in his abdomen with the sense of determined aggression in his jaw. Ray initially reported experiencing tingling throughout his body that made him feel more alive. However, he was not able to sustain this enlivening feeling and began to close in on himself with a collapsing posture and constricted breathing. I suspect that this shutdown was due to his pervasive survivor's guilt, which was immediately triggered by the experience of feeling alive. We can clearly observe how his head looks downward. To explore this guilt, I had him say the following words and notice what was happening in his body as he said them: "I am alive … I am here … I survived … not everyone did." This scripted probing allowed

---

* See *In an Unspoken Voice* for a description of this exercise.

him to both acknowledge the guilt and begin to confront his rage. Eventually, this rage led to uncovering his profound sorrow at losing close comrades from his band of brothers.*

In order to help Ray process his rage and access his underlying feelings of loss, vulnerability, and helplessness, I enlisted two members of the group to help him both contain and direct his rage. I wanted him to be able to sustain this movement and direct it into a large pillow—rather than cathartically exploding with it. Due to his deep fear that his anger and rage could potentially cause him to hurt others, he habitually restrained the impulse to strike out. This impulse to punch and destroy engaged his anterior muscles. In sensing this compelling (but unacceptable) urge, he simultaneously contracted the muscles on the back of his of his arms and his shoulders to prevent this forbidden impulse to annihilate other people. However, this neuromuscular inhibition locked up his body and buried his softer feelings in a kind of muscular "armoring."

The two group members now "took over" the restraining function (of holding back) and then helped him to contain and channel the action of striking out so that he could feel and move forward with the uninhibited impulse in a safe and titrated way. This allowed him to experience his full "healthy aggression" and contact his "life force," his *elan vital*. He repeated this directed action three times, letting the sensations and activation settle after each prolonged and sustained forward thrust.

---

* This kind of emotional processing couldn't have occurred without first sufficiently resolving the shock reactions (due to the blast explosions). This resolution transpired, primarily, in my first three sessions with Ray. However, we continued to visit the attenuated residual of these shock reactions, as these echoes faintly reemerged from time to time.

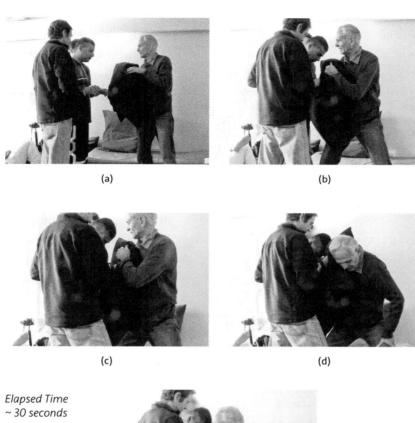

(a)   (b)

(c)   (d)

Elapsed Time
~ 30 seconds

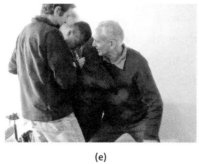

(e)

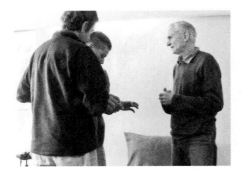

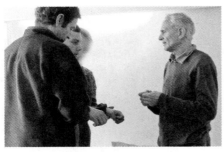

After the third time, I asked him what he noticed in his hands and arms. He responded, "They feel really strong ... in a good way ... like I can move forward in my life. I feel the strength to get what I want from my life now while still honoring my buddies who fell." This forward movement in life is the essence of "healthy aggression."

At this point we sat down together, side by side. Ray described how it was for him when he saw his best friend die in his arms, the utter helplessness and loss. With my support, and that of the group, he did this, quietly, with grace, calm, and—most importantly—dignity. Tears welled up in his eyes as he calmly acknowledged and shared his pain and grief with the group.

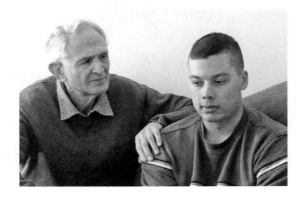

This "soft feeling" component is the culmination of an organic, six-phase, sequential process involving (1) resolving the shock reaction from the blasts; (2) imaging a future different from his past; (3) dealing with his guilt and rage with group support and containment; and (4) contacting his healthy aggression and inner strength, which (5) allowed him to, finally, quietly come to terms with his deeper feelings of grief, helplessness, and loss, and (6) orient in the here and now. Ray, who was shy within groups, began to look at me and around the room as though he was seeing the other group members for the first time. He was able to be with his deep feelings of loss yet be with other human beings. This was, perhaps, a "transitional family" for him, a link to civilian life and the world of feelings.

Some months after the session at Esalen, Ray married Melissa and they had a son, Nathaniel.

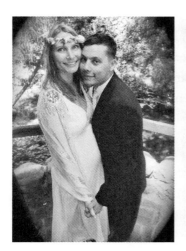 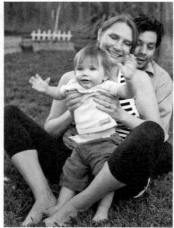

In 2012 they arranged to come visit me where I was staying in Encinitas, California, for a check in.

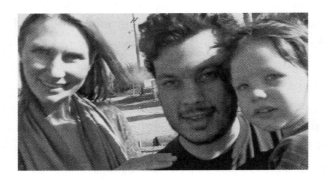

Ray described how "keyed up" he was the night before this session, due to his excitement. By using some of the exercises that I taught him, he was able to bring about states of rapid relaxation. We then did the "voo" sound and jaw movements together. He described relaxing and feeling "waves of warmth" that were also accompanied by "waves of joy."

I asked Ray how things had been going in his life. He described some of his encounters with equine therapy and how he experienced these animals as nonjudgmental and willing to trust.

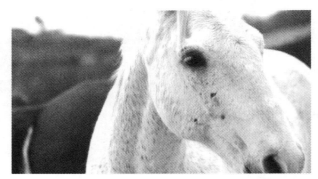

Used with permission of The Meadows Addiction Treatment Center © 2012.

I ask Ray to go inside himself and notice if he could feel the same nonjudgmental quality he did with the horses and then to notice where, in his body, he experienced this inner sense. As he began to connect with these feelings of self-compassion, I asked if he could then look at Melissa and notice what he felt for, and from, her. They quietly gazed at each other and smiled softly.

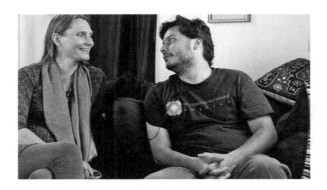

Melissa described how she had learned to give her husband his space and not take it personally when he needed to withdraw.

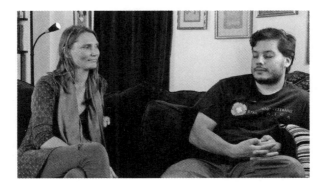

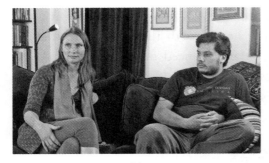

(a)

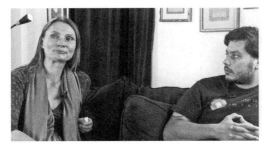

(b)

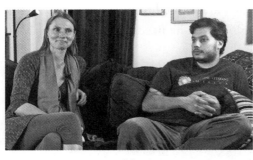

(c)

Melissa started to tear up as she described how relieved she was that they had been able to get to the place where they can stay in contact even when he needs to withdraw. This is an important skill for veterans and their families (and all of us, for that matter!) to develop—the ability to not interfere with a vet's need for "space" (and to help keep them safe), and for the vet to still maintain a connection by communicating their needs and feelings, including their need to withdraw.

Nathaniel, their son, burst into the room, and Melissa looked at him with joy as Ray took pleasure in Melissa's loving appreciation of their child.

Melissa told Ray how touched she was as he opened up more and more to her. She added that even though things can be tough, it is these moments that help keep the bond between them growing.

The session ended in the sweet social engagement of mirroring and playful interactions.

A video showing much of what is presented here can be viewed online: www.youtube.com/watch?v=bjeJC86RBgE

Epilogue and Discussion

In January 2015, former Marine David J. Morris published an article in the *New York Times* titled "After PTSD, More Trauma."[30] In this piece, he describes being discharged in 1998 from the Marine Corps and then working as a reporter in Iraq from 2004 until he was nearly killed in 2007 by an IED. After this harrowing ordeal, he sought therapy at the San Diego Veteran's Affairs clinic, where he was treated with prolonged exposure (PE), one of "the treatments of choice" for PTSD. In this form of therapy, patients are made to relive, over and over, the worst horrors and terrors of their war experiences; by retelling the story of their trauma to their therapists, patients will theoretically "unlearn" the traumatic reaction they have to those particular memories.

The event Morris chose to focus on in therapy was the IED ambush he had survived in 2007 while reporting in southern Baghdad. "Over the course of our sessions, my therapist had me retell the story of the ambush dozens of times," Morris writes. "I would close my eyes and put myself back inside the Humvee with the patrol from the Army's First Infantry Division, back inside my body armor, back inside the sound of the IEDs going off, back inside the cave of smoke that threatened to envelop us all forever. It was a difficult, emotionally draining scene to revisit." He hoped that over time, with enough repetitions of the story, he would rid himself of his terror. Instead, after a month of therapy, he began to have more acute problems: "I felt sick inside, the blood hot in my veins. Never a good sleeper, I became an insomniac of the highest order. I couldn't read, let alone write. ... It was like my body was at war with itself." When Morris's therapist dismissed his increased anxiety and concern about the efficacy of PE, Morris left, calling the treatment "insane and dangerous."

Morris also critiques PE for its focus on a single event—the equivalent, he presciently noted, "of fast-forwarding to a single scene in an action film and judging the entire movie based on that." This brief, cursory observation makes a very important point about PE and other cathartic therapies: These dramatic therapies operate with the implied belief that each traumatic memory is an isolated island, a very specific "tumor" that needs to be cut out, excised. This reified, illusory view of traumatic memory, as a thing to be repetitively relived and thus resected, dismisses the organic gestalt of body, mind, and brain in integrating the entirety of an individual's encounters with stress and trauma, as well as of triumph, happiness, and goodness—that is, within the full developmental arc of one's entire life. It is here that I feel prolonged exposure types of therapies miss the mark. And though they undoubtedly do help some, they harm others. It is revealing that there is an extremely large dropout rate of those who, like Morris, elect not to continue because of mounting distress. But let us look at a brief history of abreaction and trauma.

Abreaction—derived from the German *Abreagieren*—refers to the reliving of an experience in order to purge it of its emotional excesses.[31] The therapeutic efficacy of this has been likened to "lancing a boil." Piercing the wound releases the "poison" and allows the wound to heal. In the same way the lancing process is painful, reliving the trauma can be highly distressing for the patient. Hopefully, the freshly opened wound, according to this kind of analogy, will be able to heal. However, this may not avoid renewed infection, and unfortunately, this can happen, as Morris so aptly chronicled. And while Somatic Experiencing, the approach I used with Jack and Ray, works much more gently with procedural memories, no therapy is foolproof. Although, I would offer, its slower and titrated process has a wider margin of safety, which decreases the likelihood of retraumatization when compared with PE and other cathartic therapies. I sincerely hope that therapists using exposure methods will use some of the tools outlined here to inform and evolve their therapeutic work.

Eventually, Freud seemed to construe that the repressed emotions connected to a trauma could be released by merely talking about them; this "discharge" of traumatic affect could be produced by bringing "a particular moment or problem into focus."[32] This method would become the foundation of Freud's approach to treating (so-called) hysterical conversion symptoms.[33] By the time of World War II, hypnosis and phenobarbital (narco-abreactions) were utilized to elicit intense emotional catharsis. However, these methods were eventually abandoned because the results were often deleterious or, at the least, only short-lived. Interestingly, one of the patients at San Diego's Balboa Naval Hospital in 1943 was the science fiction writer L. Ron Hubbard, who later founded Scientology. Hubbard claimed that "clearing" (the abreacted purging of traumatic events by Scientology's techniques) was a discovery he made on his own—after being wounded in battle.[34] Not surprisingly, there is no mention of the therapy (which was most certainly cathartic) that he received at the San Diego Naval Hospital in 1943.

Next in this quasi-evolution of cathartic therapies, Joseph Wolpe introduced a graded form of exposure therapy during the 1950s.[35] This type of therapy was originally designed for the treatment of simple phobias, such as the fear of heights, snakes, or insects. During the procedure, the person would be shown a spider or made to imagine one several times, gradually moving in closer each time to the "feared object" until the charge was "bled off." Prolonged exposure therapy, as developed by Edna Foa and her colleagues at the University of Pennsylvania in the 1980s, was built on Wolpe's prototypic method for eliminating simple phobias. However, in aiming to treat PTSD and other diverse traumas, PE took on a very complex and fundamentally different phenomenon than evidenced in simple phobias. It is predicated upon the idea that after traumatic experiences like IED ambushes, explosions, plane crashes, and sexual assaults, survivors can "overlearn" from the event, allowing fears arising from their trauma to dictate their behavior in everyday life.

I believe the repurposing of a therapy originally designed for simple phobias to treating trauma, which is much more complex, may be a disturbing misapplication of these early methods.

Ray's Epilogue

Some of us think that holding on makes us strong,
but sometimes it is the letting go.
—HERMANN HESSE

A man, when he does not grieve, hardly exists.
—ANTONIO PORSCHE

There must be those among whom we can sit down
and weep and still be counted as warriors.
—ADRIENNE RICH

As we saw with Ray, there are other methods for treating trauma that are much less "violent" than PE and that operate in an entirely different way. Somatic Experiencing, the approach I am utilizing here, is not primarily about "unlearning" overlearned outcomes of trauma by rehashing but about *creating new experiences* that contradict those overwhelming feelings of helplessness.[35, 36] Ray's transformation was much more than simply unlearning or understanding his trauma response and thought process. It was about *completing* (and thereby "renegotiating") the explosive shock to his body and subsequently "melting" and then processing the frozen emotions of rage, grief, and loss held so deeply in his psyche and soul.

As was demonstrated in the case presentation, the resolution of his "stuck" shock/shutdown involved a gradual revisiting (and completion) of his orienting and hyper-protective responses to the blast. These innate protective reactions included ducking, flexing, and bracing. If we had worked immediately and exclusively with his guilt, rage, and grief, it would have been unproductive at best, or, at worst, counterproductive by potentially intensifying his shock reaction and reengaging a discouraging repetition of his tics and seizure-like movements. Work with procedural and emotional memories requires careful monitoring and tracking of the individual's bodily responses. These responses include gestures, facial micro-expressions (indicating transient emotional states), and postural adjustments, as well as autonomic signs such as blood flow (vasoconstriction and dilation as perceived by changes in skin coloration), heart rate (identified by observing carotid artery pulse), and spontaneous changes in breath.

The initial session progressed through an important sequence of observation and engagement. The first phase was to note that his gaze was directed away from me and downward toward the floor. It was important, at this point, not to compel or even invite eye contact. This would likely have been further distressing and caused greater shutdown, shame, and disconnection. Phase two consisted of my guiding him into a gradual introduction to his body sensations without permitting this experience to become overwhelming. Phase three involved *uncoupling* the tightly coiled sequence of neuromuscular contractions that were the aftermath of the successive contractions of his eyes, neck, and shoulders in reaction to the blast. These contractions were the consequence of his body's attempt to first orient and then defend itself against the shockwaves of the two blasts. This involved contractions of all of the body's flexor muscles, a reflex probably inherited from our arboreal ancestors: curling into a tight ball is the way baby primates protect themselves when they inevitably fall out of trees. As adults it may also protect against blows to the abdomen.

The segue between phases two and three was carried out through awareness work with Ray's jaw muscles and then with the guided tracking of his eyes. With these very simple awareness exercises he almost immediately felt tingling, warmth, easy breath, and deep relaxation. Phase three was elaborated over the next four sessions. By the fourth session, the startle ("Tourette's") response was nearly absent and so it was possible to begin accessing and processing his *emotional memories* of guilt, rage, grief, and loss. The final work was done in the context of a group experience at the Esalen Institute. There Ray was able, with the support of group members, to learn how to both direct and contain his rage. This contained experience allowed him to rechannel and transform his rage into strength and healthy aggression—in other words, the capacity and energy to move toward what he needs in life. Finally, this shift opened the portals to his softer feelings of grief and loss, and the desire to emotionally connect with others.

If I had prompted Ray to abreact the explosion of the IEDs with the sounds, smoke, and chaos (as with Morris's prolonged exposure therapy at the VA), it would have merely reinforced and intensified his startle response and gotten him more deeply locked in his body. Indeed, in 2014, a *60 Minutes* program showed a group of soldiers undergoing PE. At the end when the soldier was asked if he felt better, most likely not wanting to offend an authority figure, he replied with something like, "I guess so." However, for anyone who could read bodies, it was clear that he was in significantly greater distress and had been thrust deeper into shutdown.

If I had pressed Ray to try and deal with his rage, guilt, and sorrow before attending to and resolving his global startle response, it is likely that these intense emotions would have been reinforced, likely leading to retraumatization. Hence, the essential nature of the carefully orchestrated sequence of first attenuating the shock-startle response and then, gradually, with close contact and support from the group, helping Ray to access his feelings and come to peace with them. It is this sequence that made it possible for Ray to transition his attachments and vulnerable feelings to his family, as well as to other vets whom he has touched. This outreach was his new duty. Thank you Ray, truly a proud Marine, for both of your services.

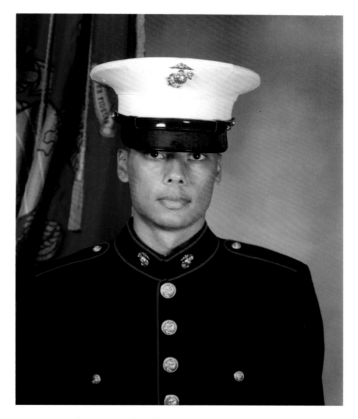

Ray, a proud Marine. This photo was taken when Ray joined the service in 2005.

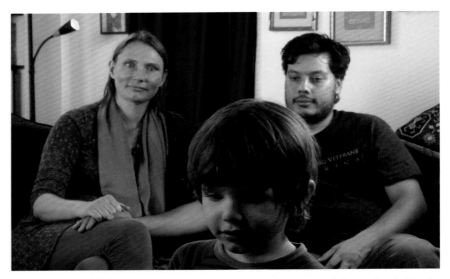

Ray and Melissa share in the caring enjoyment of their son, while Nathaniel basks in the comfort of this warm attention.

THE VERACITY TRAP AND THE PITFALL OF FALSE MEMORY

Bring [up] the past, [but] only if you're going to build from it.
—Doménico Estrada

Recall from Chapter 4 my misadventure with Laura in Mythenquai Park, where we mistook the errant children playing in the bamboo for an unnamed, stalking predator. That is to say, we were the victims of the evolutionary bias toward false-positives, toward initially perceiving danger even when it is extremely unlikely. In nature, as it was here, the consequence of a false-positive assessment is relatively minor. For this reason, we are hardwired to perceive danger, however likely or unlikely it may be.

Taking this compelling bias of expecting danger into account, it is easy to appreciate how we gauge the seriousness of a threat by the intensity of the associated negative emotion. Most simply put, the more intense an emotion of fear or anger, the more we are hardwired to presume our assessment of threat to be true, that is, to be a real danger we must react to—full out—with our basic survival responses of flight or fight. In other words, *we equate veracity with emotional intensity.* Our feelings inform our beliefs; our beliefs reinforce our feelings. This positive feedback loop, a "veracity trap," is particularly relevant in understanding the potential for the generation of spurious "recovered memories" in therapy. Furthermore, this trap is reinforced and strengthened by the strong tendency of our mind to "offer up" images that, in some way, seem to "explain" to us what we are feeling. So for example, if as a child an individual has had a terrifying medical procedure and is now abreacting the intense emotions of terror and rage, he may (erroneously) visualize this original body violation as torture or rape. This confusion can occur if his flood of potent emotions is paired with either a therapist's interpretations, or a group's collective themes of abuse. The client is likely to grab onto these leading suggestions, have a confabulated "flashback" (evoking an even greater flood of emotions), and then register this rendering as certain or factual. Since we have a reduced capacity to stand back, observe, and evaluate when experiencing intense emotions, we are easily swept away into potentially false attributions. We then become more and more certain that these things have actually happened to us, sometimes even regardless of their improbability.

These pitfalls warn us of how such misattributions can contribute to therapy's becoming harmful and destructive. The images and stories we attach to emotionally charged experiences not only predispose us to false memories but can make it difficult to move forward in life. Of course, it goes without saying that we must also appreciate that widespread abuse does happen to children; of that there is no question. And yet, in therapy, whether the memories are true or not shouldn't be the primary concern. What is critical to recognize is that the client is stuck in an engram imprinted on brain and body—a procedural and emotional memory that is dominating their affect, mood, and behaviors. So in either case, whether the attribution is actual or misconstrued, we must understand that the impact and meaning of their experiences hold truth and value. We are obliged, as therapists and healers, to help our clients liberate the vast survival energy that is bound in their nervous system—regardless of the specifics of the trauma—so that they can expand into greater freedom and peaceful grace.

The "Veracity Trap"

What follows is a familiar illustration of the "veracity trap" and its deleterious consequences in everyday life. Recall the last time you were in the throes of a really nasty argument with a spouse or an acquaintance, or perhaps watching someone else in the heat of an "out for blood" verbal duel. An unbiased witness, observing from the periphery, can quickly perceive how as the argument escalates, each person becomes more entrenched in their position, as well as increasingly threatened by the other person's perspective. This escalating emotional spiral of vehemence convinces both antagonists that they are right and that the other is dead wrong—that what they are feeling is true and therefore what the other is feeling (or believing) is utterly and dangerously false. It is this polarizing tendency to believe in the *exclusive truth* of our convictions, particularly when accompanied by high-intensity emotions, that is the fundamental essence of righteous indignation. For an illustration of the veracity effect, one needs simply to turn on AM talk radio shows or political TV channels, whether on the left or the right. These commentators exploit the power of anger to sell their political commodity as they preach to their choirs.

Let's examine a far different example of how the perceived truth of a situation, or tenacity of a belief, is frequently proportional to the intensity of the associated emotion. While we have discussed this dynamic for the problematic emotions of fear, terror, anger, or rage, it can also hold true for intensely experienced positive emotions like exhilaration or ecstasy. Indeed, this may be a dark side of religious fervor—when one experiences religious ecstasy (often brought on by group rituals involving intense breathing and movement), people may take their consensus belief to be absolutely true, i.e., to be "the truth." As a consequence, the "believers" are vulnerable (particularly when guided by a charismatic leader) to experience all the other religions (sects, groups, etc.) as intrinsically bad and as existential threats. Have we not seen enough vicious crusades and wars propelled by such fervent emotional intensity?

In summary, it is crucial to comprehend the clinical implications of the evolutionarily advantageous false-positive bias and the ways in which perceived veracity is coupled with intense emotions. Within the context of therapy, just as in religious extremism and evolutionary biology, the hotter an emotion, the more it validates the authenticity of our convictions. Hence, any images, suggestions, or beliefs that we are experiencing, along with a hot emotion, will appear to be true, that is, to be factual. "Recovered memory" therapy, involving intense emotional catharsis, often engages this same type of escalation. For this reason, the evoked memory amalgams (i.e., sensation plus emotion plus image) will frequently be perceived as true and factual, regardless of their actuality. If this is a horrific recovered memory, there is an extreme intensification of the current emotional state. This attachment to perceived truth is particularly likely when other members of a group emote their own horrors, terrors, and rage. We can also be vulnerable to a timely, suggestive hint or leading question that is offered by the therapist.* Further, with more images and suggestions being provided, the distress becomes even more acute. This iterative emotional escalation can then lead, in turn, to evoking more seemingly "true" memories. The more intense the associated sensations and emotions are, the more we become attached to the veracity of a (seeming) memory and the

---

* For practitioners of hypnotherapy (or hypnoanalyses), there is often an intrinsic suggestibility factor. Indeed, sometimes hypnosis is defined as a state of increased suggestibility. Hence, this kind of therapy requires a great deal of training, skill, and caution.

more defensive we become if this belief is challenged. These attributions can take on an almost religious conviction, directly interfering with therapeutic resolution and forward momentum in life. It is for this reason that traumatic memories must be approached from a platform of relatively calm, settled, and present (here-and-now) experience. While some of this may seem repetitious, these concepts are such a potent, and often unrecognized, dimension of trauma therapies that they can hardly be overstated.

Having said all of this, it is essential to also acknowledge and appreciate that the incidence of sexual abuse is alarmingly high and its enduring effects profoundly corrosive. Today in the United States there are well over 39 million adults (distributed among all races and socioeconomic levels) who have survived childhood sexual abuse. Obviously this is not a rare event, and it is a profoundly confusing betrayal that must be sensitively and fully addressed in therapy. Healing from this sacred wound ultimately includes the reclamation of the capacity for pleasure and intimate, joyful sexuality.[38]

On the Manipulation of Memory

In 1989 I was asked to see a young man, "Brad," who had endured a serious depression after being treated by a "recovered memory" therapist. After a preliminary assessment, she had promptly diagnosed him as being the victim of ritual abuse. Her actual words to him were, "I am sorry to have to tell you this, but your symptoms are nearly identical to those of my ritually abused patients." For the year following her "diagnosis," Brad participated in group therapy with this clinician. Accompanied by violent emotional abreactions, he recovered many "memories" closely resembling those of other group members who were similarly diagnosed.

In our work together, I introduced Brad to body awareness and taught him some basic grounding and centering exercises.[39] I then showed him how to track sensations as they emerged in his body. With these developing skills, and some calming reassurances that we would not be dredging for memories, we continued to explore his *here-and-now body sensations*. Together we learned about the many nuances of his interoceptive world. After fifteen or twenty minutes of this sensate tracking, I brought his attention to a slight arching in his lower back that I had observed. As he became aware of this emerging postural adjustment, he reported a very disturbing, fearful sensation accompanying the arching. Along with an associated spontaneous retraction of his pelvis, he reported that his genitals were "going numb." Indeed, it is likely that if Brad had been fed a leading question at this moment, a "false memory" could have easily been evoked.

Instead, I encouraged Brad to first sense his extremities (hands and feet) and then to shift his focus back and forth between these peripheral sensations (which felt neutral and even grounding to him) and the disturbing genital ones. This process gave him enough "distance," so that he was not overwhelmed by the distressing sensations. Shifting between the grounding in his extremities and the disturbing genital contraction and numbing enhanced his tolerance for discomfort. It promoted his capacity to stay focused on his body sensations.

The introceptive back-and-forth also allowed the sensations accompanying the arching and retraction to unfold. Suddenly, a clear image arose of Brad's embarrassed, awkward mother, roughly pulling bandages from his penis. He then recalled how she had brusquely dressed and cleaned his wound following a medically necessary circumcision at the age of twelve. Granted, there is no way to know with absolute certainty if this was, indeed, the actual event precipitating his depression, but I did not question the image. Rather, we integrated this new image with the arching behavior.

I encouraged Brad to continue following his protective retracting movement and to now shift his attention between the movement and the potent image of his mother's angry and embarrassed face. This retraction continued to build until it reached its full arc and completion. Brad then felt a powerful wave of release and relief. This was accompanied by tremors and a deep, shuddering intake of breath that was followed by a full, spontaneous exhalation. He was finally able to protect himself—both from his mother's harsh treatment, as well as from his former therapist's profound misattunement and misguided manipulation. This time, in lieu of the violent abreactions he had repeatedly experienced in the group, a lone tear expressed his sadness, anger, and relief. He was now able to reconnect his "body memory" with a coherent narrative, one that he was able to share with another person. Ultimately, he was able to share this narrative with a public official, and in an act of well-justified revenge (a further completion of his self-protection), he contributed his testimony to a malpractice hearing after which the therapist's license was suspended.

Returning briefly to the power of false memories to be believed as true, even when they can be factually proven to be false, let us look at a particularly sinister example of deliberately implanting false memories: Using (abusing) aggressive, high-intensity pressure and instilling extreme fear in the suspects they are interviewing, police may deliberately inject into a suspect's story some element that they know to be false (or, at least, inconsistent). Then, when the suspect is interrogated at a later time, he will sometimes tell the interrogator's version, *believing it to be true, to be his own.*

In many cases, clearly false memories have become so deeply entrenched in suspects that their inconsistencies are then used against them by prosecutors to obtain what have been in many instances false convictions. Amazingly, a significant proportion of these innocent individuals have come to believe that they were guilty. Their newly implanted false memories may last for a lifetime, though some innocent convicts do realize that they have been duped—unfortunately far too late, and then only when DNA evidence or witness recantations have definitively proven their innocence.*

This appalling use of malevolent police interrogation methods is a clear example of deliberately implanting false memories. However, as already noted, spurious memories as powerful and long lasting as Brad's can also be inadvertently implanted by even the faintest suggestion from a therapist. Sometimes the seemingly innocuous hint can be delivered as a benign query—such as, "Can you tell me a little about your relationship with your father?"—at a point when the individual is experiencing feelings that might be associated with some kind of violation. These therapeutic missteps are most likely to occur when clients are in states of high arousal, particularly when experiencing intense ("uncontained/unbounded") levels of fear/terror or anger/rage.

Vulnerability to the generation of spurious memories is also, in large part, caused by the often desperate need people have, when in a distressed state, to explain to themselves *why* they are feeling these deeply troubling sensations and emotions. This "explanation compulsion" stems from our survival-based imperative to search our memory banks for any prior information that might provide relevant motoric strategies (i.e., previously successful procedural memory engrams) to enhance current survival.

However, in therapy, our client's distressed state is calling for a solution to their *experience of feeling threatened*. This sought-after solution similarly drives them to comb their memory banks for any previously successful strategies that might neutralize similar threat

---

* See the television series *Rectify* (SundanceTV) for a nuanced treatment of this confusion.

configurations. This compelling "search engine" will grab at any sensation, image, or behavior (somatic markers and engrams) that somehow matches their present experience. As mentioned previously, this biological drive is meant to capture a successful strategy for mediating the current distress (perceived threat). However, these somatic markers keep reactivating in the absence of clear defensive and protective actions. Instead of the arousal state subsiding through effective action, the sensations and images keep reactivating greater and greater distress in a self-reinforcing positive feedback loop of escalating activation, much like the squeal of feedback when a microphone is pointed toward a speaker. (See Figure 5.1, insert following page 58.) Without the guidance of an informed therapist, this reiterative process can continue until the individual is swept into an intensifying cycle of distress, rage, terror, overwhelm, and despair. With no exit (in the absence of effective action), they are swallowed by the endless reliving of trauma.

Out of the Black Hole of Trauma

As has been illustrated in Chapters 5 and 6, the first step in guiding a client out of the vortex of trauma, and away from this destructive "explanation compulsion," is to bring down the current activation to a significantly less distressed level. The second step is to then work with their sensations so that an individual can access their incomplete sensory-motor response and begins to experience completion in an interoceptively based *action and sensation*. These two elements—relative calm and embodied action—break the positive feedback loop with its negative retraumatizing consequences. To reiterate, when we are able to stand back, observe, and reduce the intensity of our sensations and emotions, we are afforded the possibility of also selecting and modifying the survival responses themselves.

Somatic Experiencing "de-potentiates" (defangs) the disturbing, trauma-linked implicit and procedural memories through titration and the co-evocation of supportive and empowering interoceptive experiences. Together, therapist and client reduce and regulate extreme arousal states, facilitating completion of the biological defensive responses. In the safe and supportive context created by the therapist, a client is able to complete the thwarted defensive response, through imagery and subtle (inner) movement. This will often be accompanied by autonomic discharge in the form of heat, gentle trembling, tears, and other spontaneous movements. Once the proprioceptive experience of biological completion has occurred, the memories lose their intense charge (de-potentiate). They may now integrate into the hippocampal (autobiographical) timeline like ordinary memories. (See Figure 7.1.)

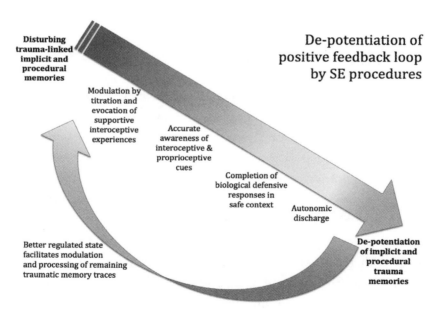

Figure 7.1. De-potentiation of trauma-based emotional and procedural memories.[40]

What follows is an exploration of the guidance needed to break the corrosive feedback loop that had imprisoned Brad during his recovered memory therapy. This review will include a brief summary of the key features of the "renegotiation" of his distress cycle. In our session, Brad and I were able to work in a more calm, centered, and gradual way that allowed him to come to peace with the profoundly disturbing "memories" that had haunted him. It is worth noting that even before his "recovered memory" group experience, Brad had clearly suffered from depression. This was his original impetus for seeking treatment. However, the depression he suffered during the year of his "recovered memory" therapy became profound and unremitting.

Brad's new outcome was made possible by first sufficiently familiarizing him with his here-and-now body sensations and restraining his compulsion to immediately identify the source of his trauma. This initial body focus and deactivation of his fear/arousal enabled him to then begin a gradual exploration of his deeply unsettling sensations without being overwhelmed and sucked into the black hole of trauma, as he had been many times during his "recovered memory" sessions. In this way, his present interoceptive awareness (of his somatic markers) allowed him to discover new embodied actions that could then be worked with productively (see Figure 7.1). Recall that with his awareness of the retraction of his pelvis and genitals, he had begun to experience some agency against his mother's awkward and painful handling of his circumcision wound. This type of somatically based empowerment could have been experienced regardless of whether the memory was from his mother's rough and insensitive ministrations or from other forms of sexual abuse. Once again, it was the stabilization of his here-and-now experience that allowed him to reach back into the *procedural* memory beneath these unsettling sensations and images, and discover the protective actions that needed to complete in order to move from distress to empowerment. This is a clear example of what I have previously discussed in Chapter 4 regarding "renegotiation."

An Untimely Confession

I must confess that I have been guilty of the unscrupulous implantation of a false memory. My personal encounter with manipulating memory occurred when I was about ten years old. I had just witnessed a magic show and was fascinated, not only with the tricks but with the magician's amazing hypnotic skills. I was intrigued by his ability to put a woman in a "trance" and to get her to do all sorts of things, including kissing the magician's cheek and clucking like a chicken. For my next birthday, of course, I requested a magician's kit. When our babysitter, Michelle, arrived to take care of my brothers and me later that week, I decided to practice my new skills. I proceeded to "hypnotize" her in the same way I had seen the magician do. I gave Michelle the "posthypnotic suggestion" that she would cluck like a chicken and take her clothes off. Counting backward from ten to zero, I prompted her to open her eyes. She looked around with a confused expression, while my brothers and I confirmed that she had in fact done these outrageous acts. She appeared horribly embarrassed, though the possibility remains that she was simply humoring us. But, unfortunately, I think not. It seemed fairly clear that my brothers and I had, much to her chagrin, actually implanted an embarrassing false memory.

In any case, the work of Elizabeth Loftus and her colleagues (mentioned in Chapter 1) demonstrates that the implantation of false memories, as well as "traumatic false memories," is relatively easy to accomplish with many different suggestive techniques. While therapists need to remain vigilant for the possibility of generating spurious memories, what Loftus does not seem to understand is the crucial nature and importance (and fixity) of procedural memories in trauma. And perhaps as well, she does not seem to fully appreciate the therapeutic implications of *how* memories are inherently in constant flux, being rewritten over and over again multiple times in one's life, as they move, inherently, toward greater empowerment and peace. The real question is: To what end and by whom are the memories being rewritten?

8

MOLECULES OF MEMORY

Reconsolidation: The Alchemy of Memory

The brain's function is to choose from the past, to diminish it, to simplify it, but not to preserve it.

—HENRI BERGSON, *LE SOUVENIR DU PRESENT ET LA FAUSSE RECONNAISSANCE* (1908)

In the 1950s, the famous experimental psychologist Donald O. Hebb attempted to describe the neural mechanisms of memory, typified with the mnemonic and well-worn phrase: "Cells that fire together, wire together."* Each and every memory originates as *a change in connectivity between brain cells*. For a memory to exist, previously independent cells must become more sensitive to the activity of others. When this entrainment happens, Hebb proposed, it is easier for neurons to communicate by passing their electrical excitation across a chemically mediated synapse (inter-synaptic cleft) to the dendrites (receptors) of the next contiguous neuron.[41]

Beginning in the 1970s, research further clarified the molecular mechanisms of synaptic transmission, most notably with the Nobel Prize–winning work of Eric Kandel. In his investigations with the

---

* This particular wording was codified by Carla Shatz in 1992.

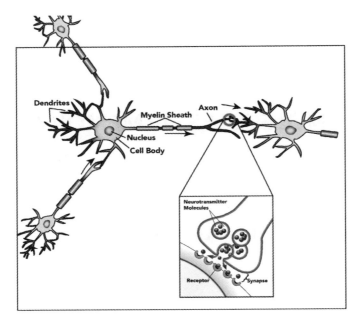

Figure 8.1. The basic synapse

simple "giant" nerve cell of the lowly sea slug (Aplysia), he discovered that the snail's reflexes could be modified by several forms of conditioning. This learning involved alterations in how nerve cells communicate with one another.

Kandel studied both short- and long-term memory in the snail neuron. Through this research, he began to unravel the mystery of what happens when short-term impressions ("sensitizations") become long-term memory traces ("potentiations"). He found that short-term facilitations involve transient changes in the synaptic conductivity between the cells, but without recognizable anatomical changes. On the other hand, long-term memory involves enduring functional and structural changes that result from the growth of new synaptic connections. These changes include the addition of new receptors at the (postsynaptic) dendrite of the next neuron. They also result in an increase in the release of the neurotransmitters used by the nerve cells to communicate. Neurons may even sprout new ion conduction channels along the length of their axons. These new channels allow them to generate more voltage, prompting an increase in conduction velocity and greater release of the neurotransmitters into the inter-synaptic cleft. Taken together, *all* of these anatomical and functional changes lead to long-term potentiation, i.e., to long-term memory storage. They constitute what is called the *consolidation phase* of memory.[42]

Some forty years after this seminal work of Kandel's, a young postdoctoral student, Karim Nader, was working in the neurobiology lab of Joseph LeDoux (the well-known researcher who coined the term "the emotional brain") and started to investigate memory from a different angle. He not only focused on what happens as a memory is formed, but what happens *after* the memory has already been created when we try to *access it* (i.e., to "remember" it). Nader knew from earlier research that specific proteins were required for establishing memories, and he wondered whether similar proteins were also created when long-term memories were later accessed and remembered. To test this hypothesis, he temporarily blocked the synthesis of the memory consolidation protein in a lab rat's living brain to see if it would result in altered recall.

LeDoux was highly skeptical of his student's research, arguing that even if Nader had blocked the rats' protein synthesis during recall, the original circuitry would still be intact; hence, the memory would remain intact as well. He further reasoned that if Nader could induce "amnesia" by blocking protein synthesis during recall, it would be, at best, a temporary amnesia. Once the protein synthesis block was removed, the memory would return since the original anatomical structure and biochemical changes (formed during the long-term potentiation) would still be intact.

In a revolutionary experiment, Nader taught a number of rats to associate a specific (neutral) sound with a subsequent painful electric shock. After reinforcing this fear conditioning for some weeks, Nader then exposed the rats to the sound without subsequently administering the shock. The rats still froze in fear of the shock, exhibiting the same physiological arousal responses Nader had conditioned in them. In itself, this "run of the mill" Pavlovian conditioned reflex was not surprising. But Nader again repeated the conditioned stimulus (the sound exposure alone), this time after having injected a specific chemical that inhibits protein synthesis directly into the rats' amygdalae (the fear center in the "emotional" brain).[43] Neither he nor his staid mentor could believe what happened when he played the sound this time. In Nader's words, "The fear memory was gone; the rats had forgotten everything." The emphasis LeDoux (and Kandel) put on the memory paradigm of fixed anatomical structures and static biochemistry was overturned by Nader's clear demonstration of the *mutable re-creation of memory in the process of recall.* Contrary to what the embarrassed LeDoux had predicted, the relative *absence of fear* in response to the sound remained stable long after the injection had worn off. Nader had, indeed, fully and permanently erased a fear memory!

The crucial ingredient in Nader's remarkable outcome was the precisely coordinated timing between the injection of the protein inhibitor and the evocation of a memory. In addition, the rats forgot *only the unique memory* (the specific sound), the one they had been forced to remember during the time interval when they were "under the influence" of the protein inhibitor. Fear that was conditioned to other sounds was unaffected, as were other unrelated memories. The erasure was indeed very specific to that particular tone. Simply put, *if new proteins could not be created during the act of remembering, then the original memory ceased to exist!*

The stunning implication of Nader's breakthrough research is that memories are not formed and then pristinely maintained, as was previously assumed. Rather, memories are formed and then rebuilt anew every time they are accessed, i.e. remembered. In a 2012 article on Nader's research, Jonah Lehrer writes, "Every time we reflect upon the past, we are delicately transforming its cellular representation in the brain, changing its underlying neural circuitry."[44] Nader's newly converted mentor, LeDoux, humbly chimed in with this apt statement: "The brain isn't interested in having a set of perfect memories about the past ... instead, memory comes with a natural updating mechanism, which is how we make sure that the information taking up valuable space inside our head is still useful. This might make our memories less accurate, but it certainly makes them more relevant to the present and future [i.e., makes them adaptive]."[45]

The takeaway message from this exciting line of research is that the purpose of the very act of recall is to provide the molecular opportunity to update a memory based upon new information. This is, in other words, the essence of not only how the past persists in the present, but how the present has the potentiality of changing (what was) the past. By changing our present-time sensations and images, the memories that are accessed will become more empowered. This was demonstrated lucidly with Pedro in Chapter 5 and both Baby Jack and Ray in Chapter 6, as well as with Brad in Chapter 7. When the Danish philosopher Søren Kierkegaard said, "Even God cannot change the past," he might just have been wrong, while Henri Bergson in 1908 had it right with the notion that "the brain's function is to choose from the past, to diminish it, to simplify it, but not to preserve it," that is, to update it. The central question becomes of how to utilize naturalistic methods to help people alter their memories and to come to peace with them.

In summary, the critical ingredient in the pharmacology of memory erasure is in the precise timing of the administration of the protein-inhibiting drug, along with the concurrent evocation of a specific memory. It seems probable that this time interval is precisely when that particular memory would also be susceptible to being altered, transformed, and learned from through the administration of naturalistic, somatic, and behavioral interventions. In these non-pharmacological approaches, rather than being retrieved and deleted, the memories are gradually elicited, sequentially revisited, reworked, updated, and learned from. This naturalistic memory "alchemy" likely utilizes the same temporal biological opportunity as we have seen with the erasure drugs. The outcome, however, contrasts starkly with that of erasure, where a gap or hole might be left in the fabric of one's recall. This extraction may ultimately weaken the warp and weave of a coherent narrative and a unified sense of self.

In the naturalistic model, on the other hand, during the aforementioned critical time period of recollection and reconsolidation, inner strengths, and capacities in the form of reworked procedural memories (which were overwhelmed or absent at the time of the original trauma) are accessed, embodied, reinvigorated, and allowed to fully complete and express themselves. Indeed, isn't this exactly the process we witnessed with Pedro, Baby Jack, and Ray in Chapters 5 and 6? For Pedro, it was when he first became aware of the strength in his hand—closing in to gather power and opening up to reaching and receiving. Such innate dynamic resources have a tendency to emerge when adequately engaged, supported, and sequenced—a vital factor neglected by the erasure approaches and by many forms of trauma therapy.

When we are able to "look back" at a traumatic memory from an empowered stance, the recollection will be updated as though this agency had been available and fully functional at the time of the original trauma. This newly reconsolidated experience then becomes the new updated memory where the (empowered) present somatic experience profoundly alters the (past) memory. *These emerging resources become the bridging of past and present—the "remembered present."* This memory updating in no way takes away from

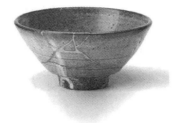

Figure 8.2. The golden bowl

the truth that a particular traumatizing event really did happen, that it caused egregious harm, and that grief and outrage may be significant components to restoring dignity and a deep honoring of the Self. From this present-based platform of self-compassion, the memories can gradually be softened, reshaped, and rewoven into the fabric of one's identity. This brings to mind the ancient Japanese tradition of repairing broken porcelain antiquities by reuniting the fragments with seams of gold. The repair of the shattered pieces renders exquisitely transformed works of art, just as healing the wounds of trauma gives rise to the natural world of ebb and flow, where empowerment, harmony, self-compassion, and dignity are restored. What could be more beautiful and more valuable?

Therapeutic Implications of Timing: A Summary

1. The timing of when you evoke a memory is critical to influencing the outcome or changing its impact.
2. For therapies that have clients repeatedly relive their traumas (such as prolonged exposure therapy and critical incident debriefing), the conditions are created whereby when the individual is in a bodily state of fear arousal or distress during the recall of the traumatic event(s), the anguishing memory is reconsolidated and may well be reinforced and strengthened, potentially retraumatizing the person.

3. When a traumatic memory is brought up in a therapeutic setting, there is a temporal decision tree. The corrective experience (the desired outcome) requires that the individual become sufficiently grounded, regulated, and empowered *before* they work directly with the traumatic memory. After this stabilization is secured, then the successful evocation of the corrective responses is dependent on the timing and pacing of the procedural memory recall. Furthermore, it remains essential that the therapist continues throughout the session to manage the client's activation, as well as their assimilation of the associated emotions.

4. Keep in mind that the adaptive function of recalling a memory is to update the memory by bringing in new, relevant information and promoting greater responsiveness and capacity to survive—and thrive in—future challenges. In terms of traumatic memories, which are by and large procedural and emotional, the key in creating a positive update of the memory lies in experientially incorporating effective, survival-based motoric responses that were overwhelmed in the original situation and that led to the failure of self-protection at that time. In other words, in the critical time period of recall there is an opportunity, not to erase the memory, but to prevent it from reconsolidating in the original maladaptive form. This is done by introducing the new empowered bodily experiences, as was demonstrated in the cases of Pedro, Baby Jack, and Ray, the Marine. Reconsolidation is a profound opportunity to transform traumatic failure into embodied success. This is the essence of effective naturalistic approaches to the transformation of traumatic memory.

What follows is an example of how the timely updating of memories serves evolution's adaptive dictate to continually upgrade our capacity to outwit our predators or to circumvent future life-threatening circumstances. A delightful BBC National Geographic nature film shows a scene where a lion is chasing three young cheetah cubs. Just barely escaping their demise by scrambling up a tree, the cubs wait with patient vigilance for the lion to vacate the premises. They then climb down, one by one, and take turns chasing the other two, just as the lion had. However, during this play period, the viewer is struck by how the cubs try out multiple strategies and permutations of their successful escape. In this way they have not only escaped on this particular occasion in this particular manner, but they have also improved their performance and the likelihood of escape in future predator/prey encounters.

Similarly, a woman who has been raped learns little by repeatedly reexperiencing her terror and helplessness. However, after cultivating the experience of agency, she learns to recognize what signals and escape opportunities she might have missed or lost to overwhelm in her original traumatic encounter. In addition, she can be guided to reconnect with various empowering, instinctive responses that can be executed in the here and now so as to neutralize the lingering sense of fear, hopelessness, and overwhelm. She is now no longer a victim but has become an empowered survivor.

It has been noted that if a woman holds out her hands and convincingly yells, "Stop!"—marking a strong, clear boundary—rapists acknowledge that they would be more likely to leave her alone. In a now-classic study, researchers asked convicted violent criminals to watch a video showing pedestrians walking down a busy street in New York City. Within a few seconds, the criminals could point out the pedestrians they would have targeted. Even more disconcerting was the consensus among the convicts about their potential victims—and size, gender, race, or age did not seem to matter. While the criminals were not consciously aware of what, exactly, was leading them to pick certain people as targets and leave others alone, the researchers were able to identify several nonverbal signals that communicated how easy the pedestrian would be to subdue, including posture, length of stride, pace of walking, and awareness of environment. In their 2009 article on the study, Chuck Hustmyre and Jay Dixit write, "One of the main precipitators is a walking style that lacks 'interactional synchrony' and 'wholeness.' Perpetrators notice a person whose walk lacks organized movement and flowing motion. Criminals view such people as less self-confident—perhaps because their walk suggests they are less fit (and probably more traumatized)—and are much more likely to exploit them."[46]

In returning to our newly empowered rape survivor (noted above), we see the critical importance of not being frozen, dissociated, and disoriented. Hence, resolving trauma through embodied interoceptive awareness, and the completion of unresolved (i.e. thwarted) procedural memories of defense, restores vital self-protective impulses, here-and-now orientation, coherence, and a confident sense (and expression) of flow. One can speculate on the similarity between the cheetah cubs' enlarged strategies in escaping predation and the rape survivors' enhanced, self-confident protection.

Types of Memory Recall and Clinical Implications

Reliving

Some therapies, such as critical incident debriefing (CID) or prolonged exposure therapy, encourage the reliving of a traumatic event, presuming that it will "desensitize" the patient to the emotions associated with that event. However, considerable research about CID shows that implementing this approach directly after a traumatizing event, when people are emotionally stirred up, actually reinforces it and may lead to extended distress and retraumatization.[47, 48] This type of repetitive exposure can lead to a compulsion to relive and repeat,[49] i.e., creating a habitual cycle which may be built on an addictive restimulating of the neurochemicals of hyper-arousal (adrenaline) and/or disassociation (opioids).

Memory Erasure

This process involves erasing a memory by blocking the reconsolidation phase through the chemical inhibition of protein synthesis. This may possibly lead to a lacuna, a gap in one's affective memory fabric. As such, there can be a loss of contextual orientation usually provided by one's associated emotions and procedural memories. Erasure provides limited possibility for creating new responses and coherent narratives, the weaving of which provides cohesion of different elements of an individual's identity and sense of agency. What remains from erasure is the likely existence of unknown triggers to unconscious procedural memories, which stay intransigently lodged in the client's body psyche, causing ongoing distress and mercurial trauma symptoms.

Renegotiation (Naturalistic Approaches)[50]

When a person arrives for a therapy session, troubled with a traumatic memory, they are either in an activated (hyper-aroused) state or feel shutdown and helpless (hypo-aroused). (See Figure 5.2, insert following page 58.)

The therapist acknowledges this memory recall and asks the client if they are willing to "set aside" the memory for a while, inviting them to attend to present (here-and-now) body-based sensations. Activation or shutdown is reduced and some regulation is restored. Then, from this platform, the memory is brought back into view, revisited, and touched into without the client becoming overwhelmed.

From their new present experience of increased containment, calm, and capacity, the individual is carefully and gradually guided to revisit the memory experience one piece at a time (titration). Each touching into ("revisiting") of the memory is followed by further normalization of arousal states, along with an augmented and empowered response capability.

The new elaborated body experience is incorporated with the original experience, forming a "new" updated procedural memory. This new memory is now reconsolidated and the old memory of overwhelm and helplessness is "molecularly replaced" with the updated empowered version.*

With the newly minted procedural and emotional memories of agency and competence under their belt, the client is guided to orient in the here and now and invited gradually to engage, via eye contact, with the therapist. The various elements of the memory are explored and shared. There is an integration of emotional, episodic, and declarative memories into a coherent narrative. (See Figure 8.3.) This process enhances the client's capacity for self-reflection and self-compassion.

The underlying impetus of the naturalistic process of transformation is our potent, innate drive toward completeness and competence, an evolutionarily prompted aspiration to succeed and persevere, as seen in the aMCC stimulation studies (see Chapter 5).

---

* Some exciting animal research supports the potency of forming new positive memories. In one study, researchers demonstrated that artificially stimulating a positive memory can cause mice (female mice, in the case of this study) to snap out of depression-like behaviors. In this recent research, brain cells storing a positive memory were labeled, and then later re-activated, after the mice were stressed. Rather than becoming depressed as they had been before stimulating the good memory, turning on the positive memory for just a few minutes eliminated the signs of depression. (Steve Ramirez, Xu Liu, Christopher J. MacDonald, Anthony Moffa, Joanne Zhou, Roger L. Redondo, and Susumu Tonegawa, "Activating Positive Memory Engrams Suppresses Depression-like Behavior," *Nature* 522 (June 2015) 335–339. doi:10.1038/nature14514.)

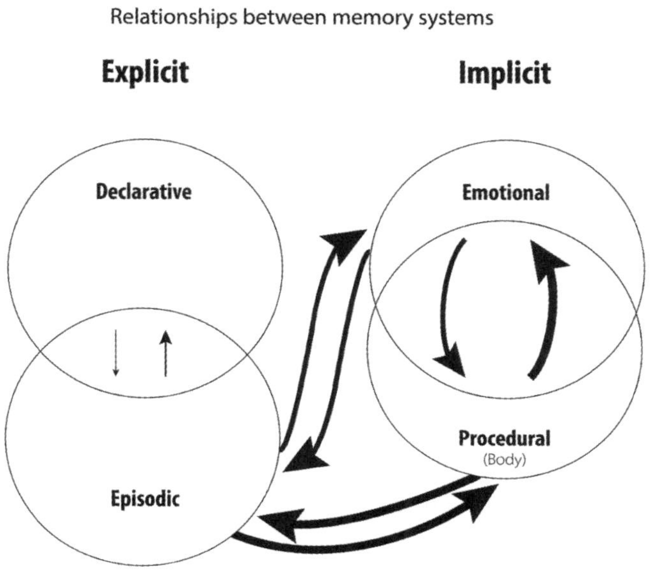

Relationships between memory systems

Explicit   Implicit

Figure 8.3. Integration of memory system

Past, Present, and Future Mutability of Memories

Over the past couple of decades, we have seen extensive application of critical incident debriefing and prolonged exposure techniques with significant contra-indications and complications. While the naturalistic means of modifying memories is now emerging as a viable alternative, it requires the careful and dedicated training of clinicians for effective outcomes, as well as validation through further research to be considered an evidence-based standard of care. The potential for a "quick and dirty" fix via chemistry is the seductive lure of memory erasure as promoted by Big Pharma and the "hard sciences." Let's now look at what this future treatment might entail.

The Future of Memory Erasure—A Fool's Folly?

How happy is the blameless vestal's lot!
The world forgetting, by the world forgot.
Eternal sunshine of the spotless mind!
—ALEXANDER POPE

Blessed are the forgetful:
for they get the better even of their blunders.
—FREDERICK NIETZSCHE

Those who cannot remember the past are condemned to repeat it.
—GEORGE SANTAYANA

We are living at a time when the erasure of traumatic and other painful memories is a very real possibility.[51] However, the "memory erasure" drugs, as we shall see, are fraught with inherent pitfalls, snag roots and hidden undertows in the brave new world of molecular memory medicine. It is an uncharted world, one rife with untold risks and unintended consequences. Not the least of these problems is that even when a memory has been (experimentally) erased with molecular interventions, it appears that the memory engram has already found its way into several different parts of the brain—a veritable labyrinth of places where parts of the memory has been stashed and tucked away.[52] As we will see (below), it is these hidden-away memory engrams that can cause the greatest problems.

Let us explore some of the inherent problems and serious ethical dilemmas associated with memory erasure, as portrayed in the prescient 2004 movie *Eternal Sunshine of the Spotless Mind*. The film opens with the two protagonists, Joel and Clementine, played by Jim Carey and Kate Winslet, waiting for the same train to Montauk, Long Island. Except for the two of them, the platform is empty. They momentarily notice one another and are curiously attracted, perhaps, as I was subliminally attracted to my first grade friend Arnold in the New York subway (though without the ambivalence). The two "strangers" enter the same train carriage from opposite ends. They sit at a wary distance, surreptitiously eyeing each other, as they begin to negotiate a dance of approach and avoidance. Clementine suddenly projects an invitation for conversation from her distant end of the train (approach). His hesitant reply of, "Were you talking to me?" is met with a derisive, "Who else?" (avoidance). Clementine continues her provocative entreaties, moving closer and closer to his end of the car (approach), while the painfully shy Joel attempts to evade her advances (avoidance). In spite of himself, Joel keeps the conversation going (approach). Their strange attraction takes on the form of an ambivalent contest in which each participant alternates between being the pursuer and the distancer. As we watch them, it seems as though these two are somehow playing out familiar roles in an agreed-upon duel, as though reading from a script that neither is consciously aware of—a script that is based upon their procedural memories of each other, as we shall soon discover.

What is not initially known to the viewer, or *explicitly* understood by these two individuals, is that they do in fact know one another—intimately! We learn that they had previously been hopelessly entangled in a tormented love affair that ended very badly. Each of them had suffered such tortuous pain at the conclusion of their relationship that they had separately sought memory erasure at the aptly named Lacuna Clinic* with the arguably well-intentioned Dr. Howard Mierzwiak (played by Tom Wilkinson). At the neurology clinic, Clementine and Joel (both unaware that the other is

---

* *Lacuna* is defined as a missing part, a gap, or, ironically, as a hiatus.

also a patient) are instructed to bring in all their mementos—photos, gifts, and souvenirs—and any other remembrances the former lovers have of the other. As they view these emotional reminders, one by one, a computer enhances their brain waves and charts the loci of the related electrical activity that is specifically associated with that emotional memory. Later, the erasure technician uses this map to fire electromagnetic pulses at those specific parts of the brain while they slumber innocently in their beds. This process apparently "erases" the painful memory—permanently. The clinic's secretary, Mary, summarizes the hoped-for outcome when she says, "It lets people begin again without this mess of sadness and phobias." And Dr. Mierzwiak adds, "While it does destroy brain cells, it is really no worse than a night of heavy drinking."

In a brief flashback at the end of the movie, we learn that the first scene of Clementine and Joel meeting in the train actually occurred, in real-time sequencing, near the *end* of the movie's plot. We, the audience, gradually come to the bracing realization that regardless of both characters' having had their painful memories erased, there remains some kind of "fatal attraction," a magnetic pull that draws the "familiar strangers" together—even though they have no *conscious awareness* of this familiarity.

At one point during the slumbering erasure process, the dreaming Joel momentarily recognizes that he may have made a great mistake. He somehow determines to focus on the word *Montauk,* as this is where he and Clementine had originally met after being separately invited to a party there. Neither protagonist consciously recalls this potential trigger word, but both have an elusive subconscious association mysteriously drawing them together. Joel, apparently oblivious to their previous life together, says to Clementine on the train, "I ditched work today ... took the train out to Montauk. I don't know why. I'm not an impulsive person." The word *Montauk* remained submerged, deep in each of their subconscious minds—an unconscious thread of their connection that had not been obliterated. However, with all of their conscious memories erased, they had no explicit remembrances of each other. They were indeed (im) perfect strangers, as though meeting for the first time on the train.*

Once on the train, however, they are strangely both attracted to and repelled by each other via their implicit procedural memories. An even deeper subterranean attractor derives from each of their individual, unresolved implicit and procedural childhood memories—the *imago* (the imprint, or engram) from their early childhood attachment relationships with their parents, as well as other childhood and adolescent developmental traumas. Most therapists have observed this kind of transference confusion in their clients (if not in themselves), who select a partner like their parent—or turn their partner into that parent. Paul Ekman aptly observed that: "It is as if many of us carry around the script for a play, a drama that we continually impose on situations when they give us any opportunity to do so. We are casting—like a film director would—people we encounter into the different roles that we need in order to replay the same script again and again. Like moods, emotional scripts cause us to misperceive the world."[53] It becomes known to the viewer that much of Joel's awkwardness comes from a childhood of exposure to bullying ridicule and the incompetence of his hysterical mother. Meanwhile, Clementine suffers from massive insecurities about her appearance, explicated through her relationship with a doll. It also becomes clear that their childhood deficits of abandonment and overwhelm (encoded as procedural memories of approach/ avoidance) are the very magnet that both draws them together and at the same time repels them, entangling them in a Gordian knot of ambivalence. It becomes endlessly snarled, pulling tighter and

---

* One is reminded of Damasios's patient David (in Chapter 3). Here David gravitated toward previously friendly "stooges" and away from those that were unkind without ever being able to remember them.

tighter, until the tension of this balled-up web becomes so unbearably taut and stuck that they both seem to have no choice but to eliminate each other from their memory banks. But alas, and not for want of trying, they must pay for their Faustian bargain.

What most of us struggle with (and what Joel and Clementine begin to learn) is that we are unable to create efficacious relationships with others while we still maintain a deeply wounded relationship with ourselves. With meager self-knowledge, we seek our identity in the mirror of the other as we once did in the eyes of our parents. Carrying all our burdens and jagged wounding, we are drawn to seemingly safe harbor and nourishment in the arms of that other—who in turn is seeking the same solace from us. Such projection onto the "magical other"[54] is a (mal)adaptive strategy that will eventually blow up, or implode in disappointment and mutual recrimination. This is what had happened to Joel and Clementine. That is, until they are finally given the opportunity to consciously absorb their projections and learn to see each other *as they really are* and not just as a substitute for the engram of their parents and their troubled pasts. Indeed, had Clementine and Joel not re-found each other they would, assuredly, have found other complementary participants to fill those roles. They certainly would still have been driven by their unresolved emotional and procedural imprints into the abyss of their unmet needs and traumatic childhoods. Without learning from our emotional mistakes, we are destined to endlessly repeat the past with whomever we are compelled to encounter. How many romances and marriages start out "blissfully" and end with the ex-lovers secretly wishing they could eliminate each other from their memory banks?

What finally allows Clementine and Joel to redo and renew their life together is getting their hands on their "memory files" and intake audio interview tapes. The tapes (provided by Mary, the scorned secretary) reveal a record of all of their experiences with each other: their attractions and aversions, their resentments, projections, and introjections. For example, in one tape Clementine says to Joel, "I'm not a concept ... too many guys think I am a concept, or I complete them, or I'm going to make them alive, but I'm just a fucked up girl who is looking for my own peace of mind. Don't assign me yours. Honest."

Joel and Clementine are initially reluctant to reengage with each other, but gradually they awaken to the enormity of their *opportunity* to use this charged intake information. They realize the possibility of learning from their mistakes and moving beyond their childhood anguish, their prejudices and ambivalences. This timely opportunity and opening moves them toward acceptance, appreciation, and enthusiasm for their potential to accept themselves and love one another *(as other)* freely and fully. It is here that Nietzsche and Pope had it wrong and Santayana got it right! Without coherent memories we don't get the better of our blunders—we are doomed to merely repeat them.

What is it that continues to live in Joel and Clementine and drive them toward each other when their memories have supposedly been entirely obliterated? Indeed, why does a woman who was abused by an uncle continue to be drawn to abusive men, even when she may have no conscious recollection of the original abuse? And if she were to regain a memory of the uncle and simultaneously ingest a memory erasure drug (while reviewing the emotionally charged memory) then, just like Joel and Clementine, she might well be compulsively drawn to perpetrators via her latent procedural memories. As in *Eternal Sunshine of the Spotless Mind,* memory erasure can create a monstrous outcome where the individual is doomed to reenact their painful mistakes *without* the benefit of conscious reflection and learning. Until they recover their once-unwanted memories, Joel and Clementine are not empowered with the capacity to form a new internal narrative that coherently joins past, present, and future.

In this same prescient movie, we also see how memory erasure can be used for malevolent purposes. Our erstwhile Dr. Mierzwiak had pursued an ongoing affair with his secretary, Mary. He later (unbeknownst to her) had her memory of this affair deleted at his Lacuna Clinic. Mary only becomes reacquainted with this history when she is caught by the good doctor's wife in the act of successfully "seducing" him once again. The doctor's wife prompts her philandering husband to "spare the kid"—and let her in on the secret of her own memory deletion and repetition compulsion.

There are other potentially malevolent uses of memory erasure that are not fictional and could very well take place, especially as these erasure substances will eventually be widely available as they find their way, along with herbal Viagra, to internet-driven black markets. Take, for instance, this scenario created by one of my students, Neil Winblatt, presented in a blog discussion of an article on memory erasure drugs. In this tableau, imagine you are sexually attracted to your best friend's wife. While drinking together at the local bar, you engage him in recounting all of the beautiful memories he has had with her. However, unbeknownst to him, you have first slipped a memory erasure drug into his drink. The next week, when at the same bar, you steer the conversation to all of his wife's shortcomings. This time, however, you slip him a memory enhancer. Consider how, with his beautiful memories deleted, he is exquisitely vulnerable to being overwhelmed by the negative ones. Hence the combination of memory erasure and memory enhancement provides you (the villain) with the perfect opportunity to manipulate the situation to your own advantage and gain romantic access to his once beloved—now despised—wife.

But let us return to the dehumanizing aspect of memory erasure. Eric Kandel, the Nobel Prize winner for his work on memory, was asked if he would want any of his painful memories erased. Since many of these memories were about his unimaginable suffering as a child during the Holocaust, his answer might surprise you:

> I have no difficulty about enhancing memory. Removing memory is more complicated ... to go into your head and pluck out a memory of an unfortunate love experience, that's a bad idea. You know, in the end, we are who we are. We're all part of what we've experienced. ... Would I have liked to have had the Viennese [Holocaust] experience removed from me? No! And it was horrible. But it shapes you."[55]

The disempowering problem with eliminating painful memories is that pain is often our most potent teacher. Maturity is about learning from our mistakes and struggles. Indeed, authentic wisdom is not free. There is a wonderful word in the Danish language that is particularly relevant to this process: *Gennemleve*, which translates roughly as, "to live something through to its completion, to remain aware of and in contact with the process, and then, finally, to come to peace with it."

With Big Pharma already pushing research on memory erasure drugs (geared toward erasing a patient's fears and phobias), there is no reason to think that they won't spend hundreds of millions (if not billions) of dollars on manufacturing and marketing these products. Predictably, Congress would be lobbied to ensure minimal regulation, and TV and internet advertising would be compelling—all in spite of potential side effects and abuses. The potential for mass manipulation for political and economic gain cannot be discounted nor brushed aside.

In Aldous Huxley's *Brave New World,* the government manipulates the population with a benzodiazepine/Prozac combo drug called "SOMA," which is used effectively to pacify the masses. One shudders in horror in thinking about memory erasure drugs used en masse, as devious politicians bring up memories they want forgotten or enhanced. Science fiction? Maybe in the twentieth century, but certainly not in the twenty-first. Memory erasure, perhaps, is also indicative of our culture's tendency toward a laziness that seeks solutions solely through drugs, be they antidepressants, stimulants, anti-anxiety or sleeping medications, etc., rather than through invoking our own creative capacity for generating self-regulation and resilience.

What is most concerning about erasure procedures is that there is no general understanding of the nature, function, or relationship between the multiple memory systems: explicit (declarative and episodic) and implicit (emotional and procedural). In fact, the greatest problem, as manifested in *Eternal Sunshine of the Spotless Mind,* is that the "success" exists largely in erasing most of the declarative, episodic, and emotional memories, while leaving the procedural ones intact, coiled in wait, ready to reassert themselves at the slightest (unconscious) trigger or provocation. We may erase a memory of abuse, but without full integration and restored agency, we will continue to have diminished capacity to respond effectively to similar situations in the future. Without this ability we may be strangely drawn to endangering situations and repetitive relationship failures that could have been addressed with interpersonal awareness and then integrated with new skills, reflection, and empowerment. Even if we are able to delete procedural memories, we might inadvertently create defenseless individuals who are divorced from their instincts, mistakenly approaching that which is dangerous and avoiding that which is beneficial. This lack of orientation, and confusion between approach and avoidance, is something that we often see in survivors of molestation and abuse.

Before jumping, willy-nilly, into a brave new world of memory erasure,* let us acknowledge that inattention to the complex mechanisms of traumatic memory could foreshadow disaster. On the other hand, bringing clinicians and scientists together in a climate of collaboration and trust could help provide a more comprehensive understanding of traumatic memory and, in turn, alleviate unnecessary suffering.

---

* It should be noted that there are pharmacologic approaches that, rather than trying to erase memories, attempt to dampen acute stress with the types of medications used to lower blood pressure. (See Pitman et al., "Effect of Acute Post-Trauma Propranolol on PTSD Outcome and Physiological Responses During Script-Driven Imagery," *CNS Neuroscience and Therapeutics* 18, no. 1 (January 2012): 21–27.) These drugs have been used (though with limited effect) when people are taken to the emergency room after accidents or rapes. Indeed, the ER itself can be traumatizing. But even then, ER nurses, paramedics, and physicians could be trained with simple "emotional first aid" awareness and deactivation techniques, along with reassurance and supportive human contact, to help people "ride through" these intense states. It would indeed be well worth a study!

GENERATIONAL TRAUMA: HAUNTINGS

I'm inclined to think that we're all ghosts …
It's not only the things that we've inherited
from our fathers and mothers that live on in us
but all sorts of dead things …
they're not actually alive in us,
but they're rooted there all the same.

—HENRIK IBSEN, *GHOSTS*

How Far in Space and Time

When I published my first book, *Waking the Tiger*,[56] one final section was titled "How Far in Space and Time." When this chapter was written, in the early 1990s, the idea of the generational transmission of trauma seemed, at best, to be thoroughly unscientific, if not fanciful. However, research over the past few years has not only chronicled the existence of such conduction but has demonstrated some of the epigenetic, molecular, and biochemical mechanisms responsible for such transmission.

In one pivotal experiment,[57] mice were exposed to the neutral (if not agreeable) scent of cherry blossoms. This neutral scent was then followed by an aversive electrical shock. After several pairings, the mice froze in fear when the scent was presented alone, in the absence of the shock. No surprise—this is a typical example of Pavlovian conditioning. However, what is astonishing about the experiment was that this same robust conditioned response was retained through at least five generations of progeny. In other words, when exposed to the scent of the cherry blossoms, the great-great-grandchildren of the experimentally conditioned mice froze in fear just as though they themselves had been conditioned to the shock. Further, when these progeny were exposed to several other neutral smells, there was no response, just as had been the case for their great-great-grandfathers. Incidentally, this generational transmission was significantly stronger through the male line.

This remarkable specificity of conditioning to one particular odor, to the exclusion of all others, has staggering implications for the transmission of trauma in humans. For example, I have worked with several second-generation Holocaust survivors who during their sessions were startled by perceiving the nauseating smell of burning flesh. This occurred along with an intense visceral reaction of nausea, fear, and a palpable dread that something horrible would happen. Indeed, a number of these clients were so averse to this type of smell that they became strict vegetarians. While I certainly can't offer this as proof of generational trauma, one can hardly dismiss the significance of this smell transmission, particularly given the results of the mouse experiment.

In an interview article titled "Trauma Ripples through Generations,"[58] Israeli trauma researcher Zahava Solomon ends the dialogue with a reflection on her own ancestry. The daughter of Holocaust survivors, she describes her very positive relationship with her parents. Her mother shared stories about the courage she and her siblings had demonstrated during that period, and how Zahava's birth had been a ray of hope, her triumphant victory over the Nazis.

Solomon concludes the interview with the statement that, "So far as I can tell, it [my parents' experience] affected me [only] in a positive way." However, "I do have a lot of qualms about aggression; I'm also quite anxious," she adds in a revealing aside.

Rachael Yehuda, one of the leading researchers on the neurobiological effects of generational trauma—and particularly on the children of Holocaust survivors—has demonstrated clear changes in cortisol levels and other physiological markers of anxiety in this population.[59] These relatively nonspecific effects could, of course, be transmitted by compromised parenting of their infant offspring. However, from my own clinical work with children and grandchildren of Holocaust survivors, I have frequently noticed and tracked symptoms of generalized anxiety and depression. I have also noted that these individuals frequently describe surprisingly specific and often horrific images, sensations, and emotions about events that seemed quite real but could not possibly have happened to them. I was able to confirm that many of these specific events had actually happened to the patients' parents, and could not have possibly happened to their children. However, the children were clearly experiencing their parents' traumatic memories as if they were their own. Significantly, most of the parents and grandparents had not initially shared these memories with their children.

Several Native American tribes tell us that the suffering of the father is carried forth for four generations,* onto the children and the children's children. Indeed, the Bible seems to concur, as in Exodus 34:7: "The sins of the fathers shall be visited upon the children and the children's children, to the third and the fourth generation." Perhaps, "sins" are metaphors for the traumas of slavery that the Jews were subjected to in Egypt and which would not be readily shed, even

---

* I believe that some tribes say four generations, others seven. In the animal model described above, transmission was followed through at least five generations.

upon their exodus to the Holy Land. I strongly suspect that many African Americans are still suffering from the residual dark cloud drifting ominously behind the eradication of slavery. In fact, the lack of adequate educational opportunities in U.S. ghettos today, as well as the subjugation and mass incarcerations of millions of black men and boys, reinforces this tragic legacy of generational trauma.

A Navajo medicine man I once met in Flagstaff, Arizona, told me that the generational effect of trauma was particularly true in the case of wars and in times of social upheaval. An example he shared was of children who were taken from their families, villages, and tribes and relocated to Bureau of Indian Affairs boarding schools. Along with this forced separation and exile, they were exposed to constant humiliation and stripped of their dignity, language, and any connection to their spiritual heritage. The medicine man also described some of the specific rituals performed for warriors when they returned home from battle, ceremonies known to help reduce the source of their trauma— *before* it could be passed on to family and subsequent generations. He then invited me to participate in a powerful ritual that had been used when the courageous "Code Talkers" returned from World War II, and which was then (in 1979) being offered to the returning Navajo Vietnam veterans. It was a critical rite of passage we would do well to learn from in welcoming, honoring, and "cleansing" the wounds of our returning warriors from Iraq and Afghanistan.

Generational Inner Knowing

The songs of our ancestors are also the songs of our children.
—Philip Carr-Gomm, Archdruid of Sussex

No discussion of generational trauma would be complete without at least acknowledging one intriguing aspect of traumatic transmission that seems to defy explanation: the inheritance of survival-based information. Specifically, I am referring to the critical, even life-saving, transmission of implicit information that can be traced back through several generations of a family's or tribe's history.

In 1990, I was asked to see a young woman, "Kelly," who had been in the Sioux City, Iowa, airplane disaster (upon which director Peter Weir based his compellingly honest 1993 movie *Fearless)*. United 232, a DC-10, en route from Denver to Chicago on July 19, 1989, lost its rear engine in an explosive blast. This severed all the hydraulic lines, making the plane virtually uncontrollable. The crippled plane tilted and plummeted downward at such a steep angle that a tailspin seemed inevitable. Remarkably, the pilot, Al Haynes, and an emergency flight instructor, Denny Fitch, who just happened to be on board, kept the plane from going into a tailspin and were able to make an emergency landing onto the tarmac of a small regional airport. Upon impact, the plane exploded and split apart. Pieces of the burning, crushed fuselage were strewn into the surrounding cornfields.* Kelly was one of the fortunate survivors. She escaped her collapsed section of the aircraft by crawling through a twisted maze of metal and wires toward a crushed opening and into the daylight.

As we worked together, Kelly recalled the sheer terror and panic among the passengers when the engine first exploded, and then again as it crashed violently onto the tarmac. In gradually focusing on her body sensations, her terror was greatly attenuated. This allowed for the emergence of the critical procedural memory of crawling on her hands and knees toward a "pinpoint of light." She then recalled hearing the voices of her father and grandfather shouting: "Don't wait! Go now! Go to the light! Get out before the fireball!" She obeyed.

---

* Footage of this dramatic event is available on YouTube: www.youtube.com/watch?v=GhSoyUWDmt0; Fitch later told his story to documentary filmmaker Errol Morris on his television show *First Person*.

Kelly next reported an image of sitting in the cornfield beside the tarmac and feeling the warmth of the sun on her face. As she experienced a relieving wash of warm sensations, she then described feeling powerful waves of gratitude for being alive and for the "life preserver" passed on by her father and grandfather. Both Kelly's father and grandfather had survived separate plane crashes (one commercial, the other military). *Both* men had narrowly escaped death by leaving the wreckage as soon as the plane hit the ground. It is, of course, entirely possible that Kelly had heard stories about her father's and grandfather's harrowing experiences, and these tales may well have helped her know what to do when the plane went down. On the other hand, maybe it was not simply remembering the stories, but having theses imprints branded onto her psyche and into her body memory.

Direct transmission of procedural memories may well serve the evolutionary function of ensuring survival in situations where conscious deliberation would be limited, if not fruitless. Along this line of thought, our nonprofit organization, the Somatic Experiencing Trauma Institute, was working in Thailand in the aftermath of the Southeast Asian earthquake and tsunami in 2004. Many of the villagers told our team that elephants and other wild animals ran for higher ground at the moment of the earthquake and before the resulting tsunami, as did many of the tribal communities. While stories passed on over a period of three hundred years, since the time of the previous mega-tsunami, could be a plausible explanation for the tribal members' escape, we cannot explain the wild animals' instantaneous "instinctual" responses by citing myths, lore, or storytelling, at least not so far as we understand the linguistics of these species.

As a biological scientist, trusting in evolution as the "go-to," default mechanism for change, my view of the transmission across time and space of traumatic procedural (body) memories is this: I see generational transmission of trauma as a necessary downside,

"a side effect," of being able to transmit and receive vital survival-based information. This information can lie dormant and then
suddenly appear as a compelling procedural memory when a similar situation is encountered, even after many generations—just as
it did in Southeast Asia's mega-tsunami or when Kelly, hearing the
voices of her deceased father and grandfather, sprang into action
by crawling to safety through the tangled mess of the crushed
and torn fuselage, thus escaping the fireball that would certainly
have doomed her to a fiery death. Clearly, these transgenerational
promptings saved Kelly's life.

Homeopaths have long recognized this kind of generational
information exchange through their understanding of "miasma," a
term referring to a cloud of contagious power that has an independent life of its own and must be treated by influencing the patient's
"energy/information field." These miasmas are seen to spread across
generations. Evolutionary biologist Rupert Sheldrake carried out a
wide array of provocative experiments suggesting similar generational field effects through what he calls "morphic resonance."[60, 61]

In one of Sheldrake's early experiments, a particular strain of
mice was taught to run a maze in Sydney, Australia. Then, mice of
the same strain—though born and raised in New York and never
transported between continents—were run through an identical
maze at the Rockefeller Labs in New York City. Surprisingly, they
learned the maze at a statistically significant faster pace. Now of
course, one could point out that everything is faster in New York.
However, when the experiment was reversed and mice first learned
the maze in New York, then the Sydney brethren claimed the edge.
If such demonstrable effects exist in biologically related mice when
learning a simple maze, then the likelihood of transmitting emotionally significant survival information between humans, across space
and time—particularly when there is something so violent as an airplane crash, tsunami, or war—seems likely to be clinically relevant.

Generational transmission is a compelling possibility that we cannot and should not ignore. And while mainstream science tends to ignore Sheldrake's findings because it does not fit into known paradigms, it should be noted that he has successfully performed many such experiments with similar results. Furthermore, a group of donors has offered a sizable monetary prize to anyone who can disprove *any* of his experimental findings. So far, there have been no takers.

For now, readers and fellow explorers, I will leave further explanations to Rod Serling and *The Twilight Zone,* but not without wondering just how far in space and time the patterns of traumatic shock truly extend and how wars, persecutions, purges, and other cataclysmic events appear to repeat, often with stunning regularity. Discovering just how these trauma-specific "information packets" are passed on as engrams—as procedural and emotional memories—from generation to generation is a vital "karmic" mysterium tremendum left for future generations to ponder.

Afterthought

The developing science of memory has made it abundantly clear that our "common sense" understanding of memory, as a fixed entity, is fundamentally incorrect. Further, when we recall the imprint (the engram) of an experience, we discover that these memories are in continual flux, changing in content and structure throughout the course of our lives—for better or for worse.

So what, then, is the role of memory in how we understand and treat trauma? Perhaps we can receive guidance from the perennial wisdom of myth. In particular, a wise counsel is reflected in the ancient Egyptian legend of Isis and Osiris. In this instructive telling, we find that the enemies of the great king Osiris had murdered and dismembered him, cutting up his body into many pieces and burying them in the far corners of the kingdom. However, Isis, empowered by her great love for Osiris, searched until she found all of the parts of his body and brought these "members" back together. In this reviving, she *"re-membered"* him.

When the seemingly disparate symptoms, the broken shards and fragments, the signs and syndromes that traumatized people exhibit are followed, they reveal clues that can be used to activate the process of healing. To comprehend these symptoms we need to appreciate what happens to the body and brain when a person is frozen in fear. Many of these symptoms can be understood to represent *disembodied parts of experience*—inchoate physical sensations that have overwhelmed these people in the past and, like the slaughtered parts of Osiris, have been cast asunder as dissociated fragments. Treatment aimed at "putting back together" these disjointed sensations would be akin to what the mythological Egyptian goddess Isis did with the disembodied parts of her husband, Osiris—she dug them up from the hidden places where his enemies had buried them. Symbolically, she then joined them together into a coherent organism; she "re-membered" him. Doing this involves gently coaxing individuals to begin to feel and tolerate the sensations that once overwhelmed them. This allows traumatic memories to coalesce, reconnect, and transform.

Finally, as Henry Ward Beecher is reported to have said: "Affliction comes to us, not to make us sad, but sober; not to make us sorry, but wise." I conclude with the hope that this work contributes, in some small way, to our collective wisdom in the understanding of how we can come to peace with our difficult memories and feelings.

Endnotes

Chapter 1

1. Engrams are the physical or chemical imprints that memories leave on the brain. For example, see X. Liu, S. Ramirez, P. T. Pang, C. B. Puryear, A. Govindarajan, K. Deisseroth, and S. Tonegawa, "Optogenetic Stimulation of a Hippocampal Engram Activates Fear Memory Recall," *Nature* 484, no. 7394 (March 2012): 381–85, doi: 10.1038/nature11028.

2. Bessel A. van der Kolk and Onno van der Hart, "Pierre Janet and the Breakdown of Adaptation in Psychological Trauma," *American Journal of Psychiatry* 146, no. 12 (December 1989): 1530–40.

3. Pierre Janet, *L'automatisme psychologique: Essai de psychologie expérimentale sur les formes Inférieures de l'activité humaine* (Paris: Société Pierre Janet/Payot, 1973).

4. Jon D. Levine, H. Gordon, and H. Fields, "Analgesic Responses to Morphine and Placebo in Individuals with Postoperative Pain," *Pain* 10, no. 3 (June 1981): 379–89.

5. B. van der Kolk, M. S. Greenberg, H. Boyd, and J. Krystal, et al., "Inescapable Shock, Neurotransmitters, and Addiction to Trauma: Toward a Psychobiology of Post-Traumatic Stress, *Biological Psychiatry* 20, no. 3 (March 1985): 414–25.

6. Bessel van der Kolk, *The Body Keeps the Score: Brain, Mind, and Body in the Healing of Trauma* (New York: Viking, 2014).

7. William Saletan, "Removable Truths: A Memory Expert's Indestructible Past," Slate.com, May 25, 2010.

8. William Saletan, "The Future of the Past: Cleansing Our Minds of Crime and Vice," Slate.com, June 2, 2010.

9. Ibid.

Chapter 2

10. N. S. Clayton and A. Dickinson, "Episodic-like Memory during Cache Recovery by Scrub Jays," *Nature* 395 (September 1998): 272–44.

11. T. Suddendorf, "Foresight and Evolution of the Human Mind," *Science* 312, no. 5776 (May 2006): 1006–1007.

12. Henry Krystal, *Integration and Self-Healing: Affect—Trauma—Alexithymia* (Mahwah, NJ: The Analytic Press, 1988).

Chapter 3

13. Antonio Damasio, *Descartes' Error: Emotion, Reason, and the Human Brain* (New York: Penguin, 2005).

Chapter 4

14. Katherine Whalley, "Neural Circuits: Pain or Pleasure?" *Nature Reviews Neuroscience* 16, 316 (2015), doi: 10.1038/nrn3975.

15. Stephen W. Porges, *The Polyvagal Theory: Neurophysiological Foundations of Emotions, Attachment, Communication, and Self-Regulation* (New York: W. W. Norton, 2011).

16. Peter A. Levine, "Accumulated Stress Reserve Capacity and Disease" (PhD thesis, University of California, Berkeley, 1977).

17. Peter A. Levine, *In an Unspoken Voice: How the Body Releases Trauma and Restores Goodness* (Berkeley, CA: North Atlantic Books, 2010).

Chapter 5

18. Peter A. Levine, *In an Unspoken Voice: How the Body Releases Trauma and Restores Goodness* (Berkeley, CA: North Atlantic Books, 2010), Chapter 12.

19. Peter Payne, Peter A. Levine, and Mardi A. Crane-Godreau, "Somatic Experiencing: Using Interoception and Proprioception as Core Elements of Trauma Therapy," *Frontiers in Psychology,* February 4, 2015, http://journal.frontiersin.org/Journal/10.3389/fpsyg.2015.00093/. This article is highly recommended reading.

20. Ibid.

21. Josef Parvizi, Vinitha Rangarajan, William R. Shirer, Nikita Desai, and Michael D. Greicius, "The Will to Persevere Induced by Electrical Stimulation of the Human Cingulate Gyrus," *Neuron* 80, no. 6 (December 2013): 1359–67.

22. Francisco Sotres-Bayon, David E. Bush, and Joseph E. LeDoux, "Emotional Perseveration: An Update on Prefrontal-Amygdala Interactions in Fear Extinction," *Learning and Memory* 11, no. 5 (September-October 2004): 525–35.

23. Peter Payne and Mardi A. Crane Godreau, "The Preparatory Set: A Novel Approach to Understanding Stress, Trauma, and the Bodymind Therapies," *Frontiers in Human Neuroscience*, April 1, 2015, http://journal.frontiersin.org/article/10.3389/fnhum.2015.00178/abstract.

24. Markus Gschwind and Frabienne Picard, "Ecstatic Epileptic Seizures— The Role of the Insula in Altered Self-Awareness," *Epileptologie* 31 (2014): 87–98.

25. A. D. Craig, "How Do You Feel? Interoception: The Sense of the Physiological Condition of the Body," *Nature Reviews Neuroscience* 3, no. 8 (August 2002): 655–66.

26. H. D. Critchley, S. Wiens, P. Rotshtein, A. Ohman, and R. J. Dolan, "Neural Systems Supporting Interoceptive Awareness," *Nature Neuroscience* 7, no. 2 (February 2004):189–95.

Chapter 6

27. Inhaling high concentrations of carbon dioxide can stimulate such primal suffocation panic, causing intense terror even in people without an amygdala (the so-called fear center of the brain). See Justin S. Feinstein, et al, "Fear and Panic in Humans with Bilateral Amygdala Damage," *Nature Neuroscience* 16, no. 3 (March 2013): 270–72.

28. Peter A. Levine, "Stress," in Michael G. H. Coles, Emanuel Donchin, and Stephen W. Porges, *Psychophysiology: Systems, Processes, and Applications* (New York: The Guilford Press, 1986).

29. Peter Payne, Peter A. Levine, and Mardi A. Crane-Godreau, "Somatic Experiencing: Using Interoception and Proprioception as Core Elements of Trauma Therapy," *Frontiers in Psychology*, February 4, 2015, http://journal.frontiersin.org/Journal/10.3389/fpsyg.2015.00093/.

30. David J. Morris, "After PTSD, More Trauma," *Opinionater* (blog), *New York Times*, January 17, 2015.

31. Lee Jaffe, *How Talking Cures: Revealing Freud's Contributions to All Psychotherapies* (London: Rowman & Littlefield, 2014), 19.

32. Freud, quoted in Salman Akhtar, ed., *Comprehensive Dictionary of Psychoanalysis*, (London: Karnac Books, 2009), 1.

33. Josef Breuer and Sigmund Freud, *Studies on Hysteria*, "Notes from the Editor," trans. and ed. James Strachey (New York: Basic Books, 2000).

34. Bent Croydon, *L. Ron Hubbard: Messiah or Madman?* (Fort Lee, NJ: Barricade Books, 1987).

35. J. Wolpe, "Reciprocal Inhibition as the Main Basis of Psychotherapeutic Effects," *Archives of Neurology and Psychiatry* 72, no. 2 (August 1954): 205–26.

36. Peter A. Levine, *In an Unspoken Voice: How the Body Releases Trauma and Restores Goodness* (Berkeley CA: North Atlantic Books, 2010).

37. Peter Payne, Peter A. Levine, and Mardi A. Crane-Godreau, "Somatic Experiencing: Using Interoception and Proprioception as Core Elements of Trauma Therapy," *Frontiers in Psychology*, February 4, 2015, http://journal.frontiersin.org/Journal/10.3389/fpsyg.2015.00093/.

Chapter 7

38. Peter A. Levine, *Sexual Healing (Transforming the Sacred Wound)* (Louisville, CO: Sounds True, 2003).

39. Peter A. Levine, *In an Unspoken Voice: How the Body Releases Trauma and Restores Goodness* (Berkeley, CA: North Atlantic Books, 2010). See also Levine, *Healing Trauma: A Pioneering Program for Restoring the Wisdom of Your Body* (Louisville, CO: Sounds True, 2008).

40. Peter Payne, Peter A. Levine, and Mardi A. Crane-Godreau, "Somatic Experiencing: Using Interoception and proprioception as Core Elements of Trauma Therapy," *Frontiers in Psychology*, February 4, 2015, http://journal.frontiersin.org/Journal/10.3389/fpsyg.2015.00093.

Chapter 8

41. Very recent studies have shown how associational learning takes place at the level of a single neuron; for example between (the picture of) a face and a location. See Matias J. Ison, Rodrigo Quian Quiroga, and Itzhak Fried, "Rapid Encoding of New Memories by Individual Neurons in the Human Brain," *Neuron* 87, no. 1 (July 2015) 220–230. doi: http://dx.doi.org/10.1016/j.neuron.2015.06.016

42. Eric R. Kandel, *In Search of Memory: The Emergence of a New Science of Mind* (New York: W. W. Norton & Company, 2007).

43. K. Nader and E. O. Einarsson, "Memory Reconsolidation: An Update," *Annals of the New York Academy of Sciences* 1191 (March 2010) 27–41. doi: 10.1111/j.1749-6632.2010.05443.x.

44. Jonah Lehrer, "The Forgetting Pill Erases Painful Memories Forever," Wired.com, February 17, 2012. http://www.wired.com/2012/02/ ff_forgettingpill/

45. Ibid.

46. Chuck Hustmyre and Jay Dixit, "Marked for Mayhem," PsychologyToday.com, January 1, 2009. https://www.psychologytoday .com/articles/200812/marked-mayhem

47. Richard J. Mcnally, "Psychological Debriefing Does Not Prevent Posttraumatic Stress Disorder," *Psychiatric Times*, April 1, 2004. www .psychiatrictimes.com/ptsd/psychological-debriefing-does-not-prevent -posttraumatic-stress-disorder-0.

48. David J. Morris. "Trauma Post Trauma," Slate.com, July 21, 2015. http://www.slate.com/articles/health_and_science/medical_examiner /2015/07/prolonged_exposure_therapy_for_ptsd_the_va_s_treatment_has _dangerous_side.html

49. Bessel A. van der Kolk, "The Compulsion to Repeat the Trauma, Re-enactment, Revictimization, and Masochism," *Psychiatric Clinics of North America* 12, no. 2 (June 1989): 389–411.

50. For a full description of this type of approach see Peter A. Levine, *In an Unspoken Voice: How the Body Releases Trauma and Restores Goodness* (Berkeley, CA: North Atlantic Books, 2010)

51. Edward G. Meloni, Timothy E. Gillis, Jasmine Manoukian, and Marc J. Kaufman, "Xenon Impairs Reconsolidation of Fear Memories in a Rat Model of Post-Traumatic Stress Disorder (PTSD)" *PLoS One* 9, no. 8 (August 27, 2014), doi: 10.1371/journal.pone.0106189.

52. Tomás J. Ryan, Dheeraj S. Roy, Michele Pignatelli, Autumn Arons, and Susumu Tonegawa, "Engram Cells Retain Memory Under Retrograde Amnesia," *Science* 348, no. 62387 (May 29, 2015): 1007–1013, doi: 10.1126/science.aaa5542.

53. Paul Ekman, *Emotional Awareness: Overcoming the Obstacles to Psychological Balance and Compassion* (New York: Times Books, 2008), 75.

54. James Hollis, *The Eden Project: The Search for the Magical Other* (Toronto, ON, Canada: Inner City Books, 1998).

55. Eric Kandel, interview by Claudia Dreifus. "A Quest to Understand How Memory Works," *New York Times*, 5 March 2012. http://www .nytimes.com/2012/03/06/science/a-quest-to-understand-how-memory -works.html?_r=0.

Chapter 9

56. Peter A. Levine, *Waking the Tiger: Healing Trauma* (Berkeley, CA: North Atlantic Books, 1997).

57. B. G. Dias and K. Ressler, "Parental Olfactory Experience Influences Behavior and Neural Structure in Subsequent Generations," *Nature Neuroscience* 17 (2014): 89–96.

58. *New Scientist,* February 7–13, 2015. http://www.newscientist.com /article/mg22530070.200-trauma-of-war-echoes-down-the-generations .html.

59. Rachel Yehuda, et al., "Phenomenology and Psychobiology of the Intergenerational Response to Trauma," in Yael Danieli, *Intergenerational Handbook of Multigenerational Legacies of Trauma* (New York: Plenum, 1998).

60. Rupert Sheldrake, *The Presence of the Past: Morphic Resonance and the Habits of Nature,* 4th ed. (London: Park Street Press, 2012).

61. Rupert Sheldrake, *Morphic Resonance: The Nature of Formative Causation,* 4th ed. (London: Park Street Press, 2009).

Index

Procedural memories. *See also*
  Renegotiation
    on the awareness hierarchy, 17
    categories of, 25–26, 37
    earliest, 94–95
    emotional memories interfacing
      with, 22–23, 96
    example of transformation of,
      51–64
    influence of, 22, 31
    as key to working with trauma,
      35, 37, 135
    memory erasure and, 158
    nature of, 25
    persistence of, 37–39
    transmission of, 166–68
    working with most recent, 63
Prolonged exposure (PE) therapy,
  115–16, 117–18, 120, 146
Proust, Marcel, 29

Q
Questioning, open, 58

R
Rashomon (film), 3
Renegotiation
    basic steps in, 62–63
    present somatic state and, 55
    SIBAM Model and, 46–50
    as therapeutic process, 43–46,
      147–48
Repression, 8, 10
Retraumatization, 117, 121, 131,
  143, 146
Rich, Adrienne, 118
Rolf, Ida, 19
Romney, Mitt, 2
Roosevelt, Eleanor, 65

S
Santayana, George, 150, 155
Schmid, Daniel, 9

Selvers, Charlotte, 19
Selye, Hans, 19
Sensations
    reducing intensity of, 131
    within SIBAM Model, 47
Sexual abuse, memories of,
  124, 127
Shatz, Carla, 137
Sheldrake, Rupert, 167–68
SIBAM (sensation, image, behavior,
  affect, and meaning) Model
    case study for, 48–50
    description of, 46–48
Solomon, Zahava, 162–63
Somatic Experiencing
    creating new experiences
      with, 118
    de-potentiation of traumatic
      memories of, 132
    incomplete orienting and defen-
      sive responses and, 101
    origins of, 31
    pendulation and, 55–56, 71
    safety and, 116–17
Somatic Experiencing Trauma
  Institute, 166

T
Timing, therapeutic implications of,
  143–46
Tinbergen, Nikolas, 19
Trauma. *See also* Renegotiation
    alexithymia and, 24
    generational transmission of,
      161–68
    history of treatment of, 9, 10–11,
      117–18
    SIBAM Model and, 46–50
Traumatic memories
    "acting-out" behaviors and, 8
    cathartic therapies and, 116
    emotional state and, 4
    fixity of, 7
    fragmentation of, 7

About the Author

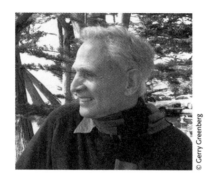

Peter A. Levine, PhD, holds doctorates in both medical biophysics and psychology. The developer of Somatic Experiencing, a body-awareness approach to healing trauma, Dr. Levine was a stress consultant for NASA on the development of the space shuttle project and was a member of the Institute of World Affairs Task Force of Psychologists for Social Responsibility in developing responses to large-scale disasters and ethno-political warfare. Levine's bestselling book *Waking the Tiger: Healing Trauma* has been translated into twenty-four languages. Levine's original contribution to the field of body psychotherapy was honored in 2010 when he received the Lifetime Achievement award from the United States Association for Body Psychotherapy (USABP). He has also received acknowledgment for his work in infant and child psychiatry by the Reis Davis chair.

For information on Dr. Levine's trainings, projects, and literature, visit www.traumahealing.com and www.somaticexperiencing.com.